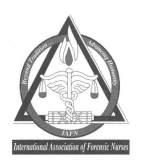

International Association of Forensic Nurses

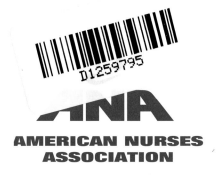

AMERICAN NURSES ASSOCIATION

FORENSIC NURSING:
SCOPE AND STANDARDS
OF PRACTICE

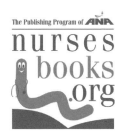

The Publishing Program of ANA

nurses
books
.org

INTERNATIONAL ASSOCIATION OF FORENSIC NURSES

AMERICAN NURSES ASSOCIATION
SILVER SPRING, MARYLAND
2009

Library of Congress Cataloging-in-Publication data

International Association of Forensic Nurses.
Forensic nursing : scope and standards of practice / International Association of Forensic
  Nurses.
    p. ; cm.
Rev. ed. of: Scope and standards of forensic nursing practice / International Association
  of Forensic Nurses, American Nurses Association. c1997.
  Includes bibliographical references and index.
  ISBN-13: 978-1-55810-265-1 (pbk.)
  ISBN-10: 1-55810-265-5 (pbk.)
    1. Forensic nursing—Standards.   I. American Nurses Association.
II. International Association of Forensic Nurses. Scope and standards of forensic
nursing practice.   III. Title.
    [DNLM: 1. Forensic Nursing—standards—Guideline.   2. Professional
Competence—standards—Guideline.   WY 170 I61f 2009]

RA1155.I57 2009
614'.1—dc22   2009008708

The American Nurses Association (ANA) is a national professional association. This ANA publication—*Forensic Nursing: Scope and Standards of Practice*—reflects the thinking of the nursing profession on various issues and should be reviewed in conjunction with state board of nursing policies and practices. State law, rules, and regulations govern the practice of nursing, while *Forensic Nursing: Scope and Standards of Practice* guides nurses in the application of their professional skills and responsibilities.

The International Association of Forensic Nurses (IAFN) is an international membership organization comprised of forensic nurses working around the world and other professionals who support and complement the work of forensic nursing. The IAFN mission is to provide leadership in forensic nursing practice by developing, promoting, and disseminating information internationally about forensic nursing science. More at: http://www.forensicnurse.org

Published by Nursesbooks.org
The Publishing Program of ANA

American Nurses Association
8515 Georgia Avenue, Suite 400
Silver Spring, MD 20910-3492
1-800-274-4ANA
http://www.Nursesbooks.org/

The ANA is the only full-service professional organization representing the interests of the nation's 2.9 million registered nurses through its 51 constituent member nurses associations and its 24 specialty nursing and workforce advocacy affiliate organizations that currently connect to ANA as affiliates. The ANA advances the nursing profession by fostering high standards of nursing practice, promoting the rights of nurses in the workplace, projecting a positive and realistic view of nursing, and by lobbying the Congress and regulatory agencies on health care issues affecting nurses and the public.

Design: Scott Bell, Arlington, VA ~ Freedom by Design, Alexandria, VA ~ Stacy Maguire, Sterling, VA ~ *Editorial Management*: Eric Wurzbacher, ANA ~ *Copyediting*: Steven Jent, Denton, TX ~ *Proofreading*: Ashley Mason, Atlanta, GA ~ *Indexing:* Estalita Slivoskey, Havre de Grace, MD ~ *Composition*: House of Equations, Inc., Arden, NC ~ *Printing*: Linemark Printing, Upper Marlboro, MD

First printing May 2009.

ISBN-13: 978-1-55810-265-1   SAN: 851-3481   2.5M   05/09

ACKNOWLEDGMENTS

Forensic Nursing: Scope and Standards of Practice has taken five years to write. It was an International *volunteer* initiative, with four focus groups (2003–2005), one lengthy comment period (2004–2005), one Executive Committee Review (2007), one survey (2007), and several communications between ANA staff and Dr. Patricia M. Speck. The focus groups were held at the International Association of Forensic Nurses (IAFN) Scientific Assembly annually and attendees were invited to participate in the development of the body of work as content was changed and sections were completed (2003–2005). The document was presented to the membership of IAFN for comment after the major revisions were completed by posting online (2004–2005). The second comment period was from the Executive Committee of the Board of Directors (2007).

After the second submission to ANA, the definition of forensic nursing remained unclear to the non-forensic nurse reviewers. In response to the question "What is a forensic nurse, and what makes them unique and different from other nurse specialties?", a qualitative survey was developed by the primary authors and administered by IAFN, with an invitation to the membership to help define forensic nursing (2007–2008). Over 800 forensic nurses worldwide completed the survey.

From the survey's results, the primary authors created examples of forensic nursing practice and revised areas that ANA reviewers had identified as needing clarification. Furthermore, they integrated case scenarios in order to compare the intersecting roles of nursing and forensic nursing. The scenarios were added to the document. This part of the revision proved to be particularly arduous and time-consuming, but its complexity, magnitude, and potential impact demanded it. The primary authors also made additional recommended changes to clarify nursing language and hierarchy for the non-nurse reader. The final document was resubmitted to the two-step ANA review process in May 2008.

The primary authors wish to thank the IAFN Presidents (2003–2008) and the Boards of Directors (2003–2008) for their patience and gentle encouragement; the Focus Group attendees (2003–2006) for their content expertise and enthusiasm about this publication; the members of IAFN who continued to answer the primary authors' questions about the scope and detail of their practice each year as the development of this document progressed; the University of Tennessee Health Science Center College of Nursing, Office of Research and Grant Support (including Dr. Mona Wicks, Ms. Gail Spake, and Mr. Chris Peete for editorial support); and Dr. Carol Bickford and her staff at ANA for expertise, understanding, recommendations, and advice throughout the creation of this document.

Dr. Pat Speck

Committee to Write *Forensic Nursing: Scope and Standards of Practice*

Chairperson (2003–2008):

Anita Hufft, PhD, RN

IAFN BOD Liaison:

Patricia M. Speck, DNSc, FNP-BC, FAAN, FAAFS, DF-IAFN, SANE-A, SANE-P
President, IAFN (2003–2004)
Immediate Past President, IAFN (2005–2006)
Past President, IAFN (2007–present)

Primary Authors:

Anita Hufft, PhD, RN

Patricia M. Speck, DNSc, FNP-BC, FAAN, FAAFS, DF-IAFN, SANE-A, SANE-P

Susan B. Patton, DNSc, APRN- BC, SANE-A, SANE-P

Focus Group Contributors:

Eileen Allen, MSN, RN, FN-CSA, SANE-A

Maggie Baker, PhD, RN

Kathleen Brown, PhD, CRNP

Ann W. Burgess, DNSc, APRN-BC

Cathy Carter-Snell, PhD(c), RN, SANE-A

Patricia Crane, PhD, MSN, WHNP, RNC

Donna Gaffney, DNSc, RN, FAAN, SANE-A

David Keepnews, PhD, JD, RN, FAAN

Arlene Kent-Wilkinson, PhD(c), RN

Louanne Lawson, PhD, RN, FAAN, DF-IAFN

Virginia Lynch, MSN, RN, FAAN, FAAFS

Barbara Moynihan, PhD, RN, APRN-BC

Cindy Peternelj-Taylor, MSc, BScN, RN

Julie Rosof-Williams, MSN, APRN-BC, SANE-A, SANE-P

L. Kathleen Sekula, PhD, APRN-BC

Deborah Shelton, PhD, RN, CNA BC

Daniel Sheridan, PhD, RN, FAAN

Sharon Stark, DNSc, RN APN-C

Deborah Travis, MN, RN, SANE-A, CNS

Melissa Vessier-Batchen, DNS, RN, CFN

Cathy Young, DNSc, APRN-BC

American Nurses Association (ANA) Staff

Carol J. Bickford, PhD, RN-BC – Content editor

Yvonne Humes, MSA – Project coordinator

Maureen E. Cones, Esq. – Legal counsel

CONTENTS

SCOPE AND STANDARDS OF FORENSIC NURSING PRACTICE

Introduction

Forensic Nursing: Scope and Standards of Practice identifies the expectations for the role and practice of the forensic nurse. It builds on the first version of this material, *Scope and Standards of Forensic Nursing*, co-published in 1997 with the American Nurses Association (ANA) and the International Association of Forensic Nurses (IAFN). The entire updated statement of scope and standards of forensic nursing practice is meant to define and direct forensic nursing practice in all settings and across all roles. This complex and comprehensive consensus document has been developed with input from International Association of Forensic Nurses (IAFN) membership, among others, and uses the ANA framework and guide for scope and standards documents approved by the Congress on Nursing Practice and Economics (ANA, 2005).

Function of the Scope of Practice Statement

The scope of practice statement (pages 1–21) describes the "who", "what", "where", "when", "why" and "how" of nursing practice. Each of these questions must be sufficiently answered to provide a complete picture of the practice and its boundaries and membership. The depth and breadth in which individual registered nurses engage in the total scope of nursing practice is dependent upon education, experience, role, and the population served.

Function of Standards

The Standards, which are comprised of the standards of practice (pages 23–34) and the standards of professional performance (pages 35–48), are authoritative statements by which nurses practicing within the role, population, and specialty governed by this document (*Forensic Nursing: Scope and Standards of Practice*) and describe the duties that they are expected to competently perform. The Standards published herein may be utilized as evidence of the legal standard of care governing nurses practicing within the role, population, and specialty governed by this document. The Standards are subject to change with the dynamics of the nursing profession and as new patterns of professional practice are developed and accepted by the nursing profession and the public. In addition, specific conditions and clinical circumstances may also affect the application of the Standards at a given time; e.g., during a natural disaster. The Standards are subject to formal, periodic review and revision.

The measurement criteria that appear below each standard are not all-inclusive and do not establish the legal standard of care. Rather, the measurement criteria are specific, measurable elements that can be used by nursing professionals to measure professional performance. Nurses practicing within this particular role, population, and specialty can identify opportunities for development and improvement by evaluating performance on these elements.

Forensic Nursing's International Context

Dramatic changes in health care and the profession of nursing have occurred worldwide during the past decade. Ethical codes developed by various nursing organizations provide significant guidance for all nurses and for nursing practice in every setting (ANA, 2001, 2005; CNA, 2002; IAFN, 2006; ICN, 2006). Evolving professional and societal needs and expectations necessitate a statement to clarify the scope of practice for the nurse. Similarly, the demand for the credentialing of nurses in specialty practice mandates consistent and standardized processes for defining the focus and competencies of specialty practice (ANA, 2004, 2005).

The American Nurses Association has responded with updated versions of the three documents that provide the foundation of practice in the United States: the *Code of Ethics for Nurses with Interpretive Statements* (2001), *Nursing's Social Policy Statement, 2nd Edition* (2003), and *Nursing: Scope and Standards of Practice* (2004). The Canadian Nurses Association and the Canadian Federation of Nurses Unions have affirmed similar changes with the adoption of the *Joint Position Statement Scopes of Practice* (2006) and *Advanced Nursing Practice: A National Framework* (2008). Documents such as the Canadian Nurses Association's *Framework for the Practice of Registered Nurses in Canada* (2007), Australia's National Nursing & Nursing Education Taskforce's *A National Specialisation Framework for Nursing and Midwifery* (2006), ANA's *Nursing: Scope and Standards* of *Practice* (2004), and the International Council of Nurses' position statement *Scope of Nursing Practice* (2004) delineate the boundaries of professional nursing practice and provide a framework within which nursing specialties globally can establish role expectations across all settings, including practice, education, administration, and research. The organization and content of these documents, as well as the expansion and evolution of the nursing specialty internationally (Schober & Affara, 2006), have necessarily altered the format and content of the scope and standards of forensic nursing practice.

Forensic Nursing: Scope and Standards of Practice defines and comprehensively describes forensic nursing as a specialty and provides direction for further progress and recognition internationally. Recognized as a nursing specialty in 1995 by the ANA, forensic nursing represents the response of nurses to the rapidly changing healthcare environment and to the global challenges of caring for victims and perpetrators of intentional and unintentional injury.

The scope of forensic nursing practice exists within flexible boundaries across diverse settings and populations. Forensic nurses care for individuals, families, and communities whose status or care is, in part, determined by legal or forensic issues. These patients are encountered in a variety of settings including healthcare, educational, legal, legislative, and scientific systems.

The practice of all professional nurses now includes many of the concepts previously deemed unique to the forensic nursing specialty, including violence, prevention of injury, victimization, abuse, and exploitation. Today, nurses in any country, setting, or system are expected to plan for the care of a patient who has been injured through intentional or unintentional acts that involve violence and victimization.

As the body of knowledge and skill sets identified as unique to forensic nursing expands, so does the practice of forensic nursing. The specialty's scope statement and standards of practice are intended to serve as a foundation for legislation and regulation of forensic nursing, along with the development of institutional policies and procedures for those settings in which forensic nurses practice. Given rapid changes in healthcare trends and technologies, the standards in this document are intended to be dynamic and futuristic, allowing flexibility in response to emerging issues and practices of forensic nursing.

Additional Content

For a better appreciation of the historical and professional context under-lying *Forensic Nursing: Scope and Standards of Practice,* the content of *Scope and Standards for Forensic Nurse* (1997) has been reproduced in Appendix A (starting on page 57) and is indexed with the current content of this edition. That 1997 publication was the immediate predecessor to this current edition. Its content is not current and is of historical significance only.

Scope of Forensic Nursing Practice

Function of the Scope of Practice Statement

The scope of practice statement (pages 1–21) describes the "who", "what", "where", "when", "why" and "how" of nursing practice. Each of these questions must be sufficiently answered to provide a complete picture of the practice and its boundaries and membership. The depth and breadth in which individual registered nurses engage in the total scope of nursing practice is dependent upon education, experience, role, and the population served.

Overview of Forensic Nursing

Forensic nursing is a multifaceted and complex practice specialty characterized by responsibilities, functions, roles, and skills that have been derived from general nursing practice, yet also developed in accordance with the distinctive practice environments and populations of forensic nursing. Forensic nursing practice, concerned primarily with the victims and perpetrators of trauma, their families, communities, and the systems that respond to them, may include but is not limited to:

- Assessment, diagnosis, planning, implementation, evaluation of, and scientific inquiry about human, program, and system responses to injury and interventions following injury to individuals, communities, cultures, and environments.

- Identification of the pathology of intentional or unintentional injury in those living and deceased.

- Collection and analysis of evidentiary material.

- Participation in the generation, dissemination, and utilization of evidence-based research in forensic nursing practice delivered to patients, communities, and systems.

- Utilization of formative and summative evaluation processes in forensic nursing roles and environments internationally.

- Administration, organization, and coordination of the forensic nursing role in programs, systems, and environments where forensic nurses practice.

- Involvement and influence in both internal and external systems where professional and societal regulation of forensic nursing practice impacts public health and safety.

- Development and support of local, regional, and global policy and public health as it relates to injury and the prevention of injury in a variety of cultures and communities.

- Promotion of and accountability to the ethical paradigms within forensic nursing.

- Development and implementation of professional and community education programs of interest to forensic nurses that address prevention and interventions in primary, secondary, and tertiary settings.

- Development and promotion of the interprofessional collaboration between the forensic nurse and others in all roles and practice environments.

Definition and Evolution of Forensic Nursing

The original definition of forensic nursing was "the application of nursing process to public or legal proceedings" (Lynch, 1990). The foundation of forensic nursing practice is the rich bio-psycho-social-spiritual education of registered nurses, and uses the nursing process to diagnose and treat victims and perpetrators of trauma, their families, communities, and the systems that respond to them.

Forensic nursing focuses on the identification, management, and prevention of intentional and unintentional injuries in a global community. Forensic nurses collaborate with agents in healthcare, social, and legal systems to investigate and interpret clinical presentations and pathologies by evaluating physical and psychological injury, whether intentional or unintentional; describing the scientific relationships of the injury and evidence; and interpreting the associated influencing factors.

Forensic nurses integrate forensic and nursing sciences in their assessment and care of victims and perpetrators of physical, psychological, or social trauma. Privacy, respect, and dignity characterize the services that forensic nursing provides to those affected by crime, trauma, and intentional harm. Forensic nurses are also strong advocates for minimum standards of assessment, evidence collection, and reporting of crime.

The current definition of forensic nursing adopted by the International Association of Forensic Nurses (2008) states: *Forensic nursing is the practice of nursing globally when health and legal systems intersect.*

Forensic Nursing Practice within Intersecting Systems

Forensic nurses provide care throughout the domains of nursing practice, education, research, and consultation (ANA & IAFN, 1997; IAFN, 2004). Furthermore, forensic nurses practice independently and collaboratively as needed in various settings whenever and wherever health and legal issues intersect. Forensic nurses interact with other systems in healthcare, community, and legal environments, including:

- Hospital and pre-hospital settings and clinics
- Legal or investigative arenas
- Commercial and not-for-profit enterprises, governments
- Educational, industrial, and correctional institutions

The systems in which forensic nurses practice vary depending on location, funding sources, community standards, and legal influences, and include:

- Healthcare (hospitals, surgery centers, community clinics)
- Investigative (medical examiner, law enforcement offices)
- Criminal justice (district attorney, public defender offices),
- Correctional (jails, prisons, and detention centers)
- Government (military, local, state, provincial, and federal agencies)

In addition, forensic nurse entrepreneurs establish businesses that focus on their forensic nursing practice and consultation expertise. Forensic nursing practice settings are evolving and increasing in number and variety.

The *core* of forensic nursing specifies the definitions, roles, behaviors, and processes inherent in forensic nursing practice. The *boundaries* of forensic nursing are both internal and external, with sufficient resilience to change in response to societal needs and demands. The *intersections* reflect overlap in boundaries for the forensic nurse with other professional groups by virtue of nursing's unique application of a common body of knowledge, environment, and focus. *Specialization* in forensic nursing incorporates a multitude of sub-specialty areas specific to the forensic health needs of patients in communities and across settings, populations, and systems.

Focus of Practice of Forensic Nurses

Forensic nurses are among the most diverse groups of clinicians in the nursing profession with respect to patient populations served, practice settings, and forensic and healthcare services provided. Yet all forensic nurses share skills and a body of knowledge related to the identification, assessment, and analysis of forensic patient data. They all apply a unique combination of processes rooted in nursing science, forensic science, and public health to care for patients.

Forensic nurses care for and treat individuals, families, communities, and populations in systems where intentional and unintentional injuries occur. These include but are not limited to patients who have been:

- Victims or perpetrators of interpersonal violence (e.g., child abuse, intimate partner abuse and assault, rape, gang violence, and government policy or legislation related to the violence),

- Victims or perpetrators of man-made catastrophe (e.g., automobile accidents, acts of terrorism), and

- Victims of natural causes of trauma and population evacuation (e.g., seismic or weather-related disasters).

Forensic nurses address the forensic healthcare needs of vulnerable and often disadvantaged patient populations (e.g., children, individuals with congenital and developmental handicaps, residents of nursing homes, psychiatric patients, and individuals who are addicted, homeless, or incarcerated). Forensic nurses also respond to community forensic and healthcare needs by concentrating on programmatic and systems change in the event of threats to public health and safety (e.g., reacting to environmental hazards with holistic death and mass-casualty incident investigations, forensic nursing programs and education, and policy and program development and legislation) where patients are affected by legal systems.

Patient populations cared for by forensic nurses are among the most vulnerable, disparaged, and disadvantaged in society. Forensic populations need social and legal systems to collaborate with health care to provide solutions for the identification and prevention of intentional and unintentional injury to individuals, families, communities, and social systems. Forensic nurses have both fundamental and specialized nursing knowledge and skills, including an understanding of the health-care, social, and legal systems that incorporates knowledge about forensic and public health science. Forensic nurses collaborate with agents in health, social, governmental, and legal systems to investigate and interpret clinical presentations and pathologies. Forensic nurses accomplish this by evaluating physical and psychological injury, whether intentional and unintentional, describing the scientific relationships of the injury and evidence, and interpreting the factors that influence them. Forensic nurses are experts across practice settings.

A key domain in forensic nursing practice is that of responding to the trauma of sexual assault and abuse and intervening through actions in systems to mitigate the impact of sexual violence on individuals, families, communities, and society. Forensic nurses provide care for victims of sexual assault in a variety of settings, including emergency departments or clinics (Ledray, 1999). The forensic nurse who has completed special education as a *sexual assault nurse examiner* (SANE) is an expert in history taking, assessment, treatment of trauma response and injury, documentation and collection of evidence and its management, emotional and social support required during a post-trauma evaluation and examination, and the documentation of injury and testimony required to bring such cases through the legal system (Speck & Peters, 1999). Unlike the nurse in the emergency room or clinic, the SANE is versed in the use of cutting-edge technology and techniques related to nursing assessment.

Another distinctive aspect of the SANE role is the use of a humane and legally objective approach that integrates advocacy and observation, evidentiary collection, mitigation of and protection against adverse health outcomes, including vicarious trauma, and location of community resources to support the victim. Accordingly, the SANE will have education and certification that reflects specialized knowledge about legal systems, evidence and ethical parameters, pathophysiology and injury and potential for injury, reproductive health, epidemiology, and technology and psychology associated with sexual assault, along with specialized training about the unique victim or offender population served.

The SANE role comes together most clearly in the medical assessment and treatment of the patient. While this is identical in terms of general nursing care, (e.g., assessment, planning, intervention, and evaluation), the SANE will also be responsible for representing the forensic nurse's encounter to the courts and society. This may include not only the evaluation and treatment of the patient's health status and bio-psycho-social-spiritual responses, but the health and forensic assessment, including history taking, evidence collection, and evidentiary outcomes. It will also include the systems response to the sexual assault in the courts and the community at large.

Evolution of Forensic Nursing

These key events in the development of forensic nursing highlight critical steps in the formalization of forensic nursing:

- In 1948, Article V in the Universal Declaration of Human Rights declared that "No one shall be subjected to torture or to cruel, inhuman or degrading treatment or punishment" (United Nations, 1948).

- In 1984 the U.S. Surgeon General identified violence as a public health issue, and healthcare providers as key agents in ameliorating the effects of violence in our communities (Koop, 1986).

- In 1991 AACN published a position paper stating that violence against women is a nursing practice issue (AACN, 1991).

- In 1991, Virginia Lynch's master's thesis conceptualized the "forensic nurse" (IAFN, 2008).

- In 1992 the International Association of Forensic Nurses was established as the first professional nursing organization for forensic nurses (IAFN, 2008).

- In 1995, ANA recognized forensic nursing as a specialty (IAFN, 2006).

These milestones led forensic nurses to recognize their important roles in identification, management, and prevention of intentional and unintentional injuries in a global community. In addition, forensic nursing has traditionally claimed a role in the assessment and care of perpetrators of crime, trauma, and intentional harm, particularly those whose mental or emotional disorder is related to the commission of crimes.

IAFN supports the forensic nurse in the development of international professional networks, the recognition of and expansion of the unique aspects of forensic nursing practice, establishment of scope and standards of forensic nursing practice, and creation of credentialing processes for forensic nurses. In addition, forensic nurses assist in the creation and dissemination of new and existing evidence-based knowledge of interest to forensic nurses, encourage collaboration among nurses and specialty practices, and promote interprofessional collaboration.

For example, the roles of registered nurses providing basic or advanced nursing health care to populations of clients in correctional settings are primarily determined by the settings in which they practice and the healthcare needs of their patients. Specialized knowledge for correctional nurses includes policies and procedures aimed at meeting specific primary healthcare needs of their patients while satisfying the need for security and safety. The correctional nurse is responsible for promoting health, preventing illness, restoring health, and alleviating suffering of those in prisons, jails, and other forms of custody. The forensic nurse in a corrections setting, on the other hand, will have the knowledge and basic skills of the correctional nurse, but will deliver care through competencies defined by advanced knowledge of clinical pathology related to criminality, incorporation of specific assessment tools to plan care for individuals and populations, and knowledge of injury assessment and prevention for correctional populations (Mason & Mercer, 1996; Shives, 2008).

Whatever the practice setting, the forensic nurse integrates knowledge of criminal justice, victimization, and impact of secure environments in the planning and implementation of systems to manage injury, manipulation, victimization, and trauma in correctional settings. The forensic nurse implements evidence-based practice through specialized knowledge in the detection of malingering, identification of different etiologies of self-mutilation and other forms of self harm, and negotiation of space and logistics in the management of violence and group behavior in secure settings. Specialized knowledge of the risk of boundary violations among staff and patients, along with the identification and management of such incidents, is another area of forensic nursing in correctional settings.

Practice Characteristics and Skills of Forensic Nurses

Forensic nurses provide direct services to individuals, families, communities, and populations; they affect the systems in which they function.

In addition, forensic nurses provide consultative services to nursing, medical, social, and other healthcare and legal agencies and the professionals in those agencies. The forensic nurse also provides factual and expert court testimony in areas dealing with both intentional and unintentional injury of the living or deceased.

Forensic nurses involved in death investigation bring nursing skills of observation, data collection, and analysis to the determination of manner and cause of death. The object of the forensic nurse in this setting is to advocate for the patient (the deceased) through the application of nursing skills and knowledge. While many professionals are involved in death investigation, the forensic nurse who is also a death investigator brings to any consideration of the deceased a holistic bio-psycho-social-spiritual approach, which can include the relationships the nurse ihas been able to establish with surviving family and others during investigations. Forensic nurses have an obligation to consider health promotion beyond the present investigation using the outcomes of death. The forensic nurse investigating death promotes health among colleagues, families, and communities of the deceased through the manner and tone of investigation. The forensic nursing role includes preservation of dignity, caring, and protection of rights even after death.

The forensic nurse develops and evaluates programs of care related to intentional and unintentional injury, crime, victimization, violence, abuse, and exploitation at the individual, community, state, province, district, regional, national, and international levels.

For example, the registered nurse practicing in a risk management department in hospital settings develops protocols for the collection of data and responses to indicators of patient or staff risk in healthcare settings, including injuries and other issues related to patient safety. In contrast, the forensic nurse working in a healthcare setting investigates using forensic nursing expertise (e.g., knowledge of investigation, evidence, intentional and unintentional injury) in the investigation of injury and trauma and criminality as these items relate to specific populations, such as the elderly and disabled (Sheridan, 2004) or the unexpected deceased.

While the forensic nurse and the risk management nurse collaborate across legal, social, and healthcare systems to provide evidence-based data that support solutions to risk, the forensic nurse has special expertise in cases relevant to a legal tort, such as but not limited to murder, rape, or abuse. The forensic nurse has specialized education in the identification of indicators of criminal activity and risk for injury, and the ability to distinguish intentional from unintentional trauma or injury, not available to the risk management nurse. While a risk management nurse would focus on the epidemiological trail of a virus or bacterium in an open system, the forensic nurse would focus on the evidence of intentional harm by individuals or groups that contribute to infection spread or epidemic, i.e., terrorist contamination. These nurses may work in collaboration, or the forensic nurse may be the designated investigator in the healthcare system when intentional harm is suspected; additionally, the forensic nurse can serve in a consultant role to the institution when intentional harm is suspected (e.g., unexpected death). The forensic nurse would also make recommendations to mitigate the opportunity for intentional harm in systems that will implement recommended changes as a response to risk.

Another example is the psychiatric nurse who applies knowledge of psychiatric principles and nursing theory to the care of persons with psychological or mental disorder in acute care and community-based settings (Shives, 2008). The psychiatric nurse may encounter patients who, by virtue of their emotional or mental disorder, commit or are likely to commit crimes or trauma against another or themselves. The forensic nurse in psychiatric settings has specialized knowledge and competencies in the assessment, care, and evaluation of individuals with mental disorders as they relate to criminal behavior. The forensic nurse will apply principles of forensic psychiatry and nursing to the clinical evaluation for competency and in the assessment and treatment of individuals and groups with crime-related mental disorders. The forensic nurse is a specialist in the care of the mentally disordered in secure settings, refining the care of such cases as self-injurious behavior and increased risk of victimization in secure settings (Mason & Mercer, 1996). The forensic nurse implements specialized instrumentation for the prediction of violence, assessment of self-harm risk, and determination of competency. The forensic nurse in this role has formal graduate nursing education with emphasis on forensic nursing care and interpersonal skills in systems responding to psychological trauma and abuse, neuropathology and criminology, and role transitions in victims and aggressors, where forensic nursing skills are practiced in secure settings and with the criminally mentally disordered.

Individual forensic nursing practice clearly differs according to both the nurse's experience and educational preparation and the characteristics of the patient population being served. Other major factors include the cultural, social, and legal systems in the forensic nursing practice setting.

This section has described the extensive range of forensic nursing practice. The following list conveys a similarly significant diversity of skills of the forensic nurse:

- Application of public health and forensic principles to the registered nursing practice, including bio-psycho-social-spiritual aspects of forensic nursing care in the scientific investigation/evaluation, diagnosis, treatment, and prevention of trauma and/or death of victims and perpetrators, including the measurement of outcomes and outputs of the practice.

- Development and implementation of systems relevant to forensic nursing, including development of systems that care for individuals, families, and communities as it relates to injury, both intentional and unintentional, to the care of individuals, families, communities or populations involved with criminal justice systems, and to measure the quality and safety outcomes.

- Development of quality forensic nursing care strategies through evidence-based practice and inquiry that target prevention of injury, both intentional and unintentional.

- Development, analysis, and implementation of health policy relevant to forensic nurses and forensic populations in forensic settings.

- Development and implementation of ethically sound, evidence-based, and culturally relevant processes within forensic nursing settings and systems.

- Development, analysis, reporting, and dissemination of relevant forensic data, evidence-based outcomes, and outputs.

- Identification, collection, and organization of data relevant to forensic nurses.

- Provision of testimony, both fact and expert, in judicial settings, competency hearings, and other venues.

- Design, evaluation, reporting, implementation, and dissemination of evidence-based and peer-reviewed research relevant to forensic nurses.

- Analysis of outcomes and influence in justice systems and on legislation that pertains to forensic nursing practice and healthcare quality, safety, outcomes, and outputs.

- Consultation with nursing practice communities and the interprofessional communities of medicine, legal systems, governments, and their agents.

- Interprofessional collaboration with justice, political and social systems, and the individuals who work in those systems.

- Quality education of various disciplines regarding forensic nursing practice.

- Leadership, administration, and management within forensic and healthcare settings.

- Evidence-based investigative and forensic interviewing.

- Forensic medical interviews for the purpose of diagnosis, treatment, and/or referral.

- Evaluation of crime scenes and trauma within settings relevant to the forensic nurse.

- Analysis of forensic healthcare quality through continuous review processes.

- Provision of evidence-based and safe direct patient care related to injury, crime, victimization, violence, abuse, and exploitation.

- Provision of evidence-based and safe forensic mental health care.

- Collection and preservation of forensic evidence.

- Integration of evidence-based forensic nursing practice to improve care of the forensic patient.

- Creation and implementation in forensic nursing systems and environments to improve the quality of forensic patient care, safety, and outcomes.

Educational Preparation and Credentialing of the Forensic Nurse

Historically, registered nurses have refined and developed their forensic nursing skills through clinical practice and continuing education. Today, there are five primary routes for preparation in forensic nursing (Burgess, Berger, & Boersma, 2004):

1. *Continuing education coursework* - Nurses can gain additional skills and knowledge about topics of interest to forensic nurses through continuing education courses (CEU).

2. *Certificate programs* - These include content relevant to the forensic nurse, set entrance requirements, and often provide clinical internships that result in a certificate detailing the completion of course work.

3. *Undergraduate nursing education* - Undergraduate academic programs in accredited schools of nursing offer electives, minors, or concentrations in forensic nursing that can contribute to a degree in nursing.

4. *Graduate nursing education* - The knowledge and skills acquired in baccalaureate and pre-licensure nursing programs are enhanced in formal graduate study. Following matriculation and completion of the forensic core content and prescribed forensic clinical experiences, the forensic nurse receives a master's or doctoral degree in the specialty of nursing.

5. *Post-doctoral education or fellowships* - The specific content and skills acquired in the terminal nursing degree programs are enhanced by formal forensic nursing core content and prescribed forensic clinical experiences. The programs may award diplomas.

Universities, schools of nursing, community colleges, and continuing education providers offer formal education opportunities for the specialty called forensic nursing at all academic levels. Entry-level schools of nursing offer introductory classes as electives. Accredited academic institutions offer degrees and certificates at graduate levels. Some forensic nursing education is provided by state and local government agencies, as well as by entrepreneurs. IAFN has published core domains, content, and performance measures in an outline of the curriculum for nursing educators and forensic nurses in practice (2004).

The forensic nurse brings all of the expertise of the professional nurse to the practice of forensic nursing. Entry-level practice requires completion of a basic nursing program leading to licensure as a registered nurse. Forensic nursing education focuses on injury and outcomes unique to forensic patients involved with the legal system either as victims or perpetrators or both. These areas include unique forensic terminology; intentional and unintentional injury; prevention; identification, diagnosis, treatment, and management of patients who include individuals, families, communities, and systems; psychology and psychopathology; and victimology. The principles of forensic nursing education are rooted in nursing and borrowed from public health and forensic science (Speck, 2000). Forensic nursing practice is summarized in the concepts of Wounding and Healing, Ethics, and Evidence, coupled with a fundamental understanding of the law and Legal processes (WHEEL); these principles are essential to the comprehensive practice of forensic nursing (Speck, 2000).

A forensic nurse has a lifelong commitment to learning which is necessary to remain current in clinical practice and legal issues that bear on the practice of the forensic nurse. Continuing education is required by many state or provincial governments to maintain licensure and certification. Education that is current and reflects evidence-based practice is necessary to ensure safe healthcare delivery and advocacy for patients and employers. Annual conferences, special forensic nursing interest group meetings, and educational programs and scientific publications serve as educational resources for practitioners at all levels of education, and document experience in the forensic nursing specialty. Issues such as differences in judicial processes among local, state, provincial, regional, national, and international venues; dissemination of advances in forensic science and forensic nursing science; and the evolutionary revisions to healthcare standards pose educational challenges to the forensic nurse of the future.

Forensic nurses demonstrate competency to the public through recognition and pursuit of excellence in practice. Credentialing, such as portfolio-building or certification in forensic nursing, is considered a priority for the specialty and is based on the identification of practice competencies and skills reflective of evidence-based practice. The forensic nurse demonstrates expertise in a forensic nursing role through credentialing designed to recognize clinical experience, knowledge, and heuristic practice wisdom. The forensic nurse acquires and maintains the credentials made available through certifying bodies of the forensic specialty and contributes to the evidence-based knowledge, standards, and criteria for specialty certification.

Certification offers tangible recognition of professional achievement in a defined functional or clinical area of nursing, such as forensic nursing. Through processes like portfolio-building or through examination for certification, forensic nurses earn credentials that are recognized within the profession and to consumers of the professional forensic nursing practice. The portfolio process for credentialing includes education, clinical hours of practice, peer evaluation of clinical competency, and demonstration of theoretical knowledge.

Levels of Forensic Nursing Practice

There are two levels of practice: basic and advanced.

Basic Forensic Nursing Practice

Basic forensic nursing is practiced by registered nurses who have knowledge and skills necessary for a specific role in forensic nursing, such as sexual assault nurse examiner (SANE). Basic forensic nursing practice is considered generalist and is guided by forensic nursing protocols for specific forensic populations of patients. Basic forensic nurses achieve specialized competencies through training programs, continuing education, and certification programs. Most generalists practicing basic forensic nursing are prepared for their nursing career at the diploma, associate degree, and bachelor's degree level.

For instance, a generalist forensic nurse specializing as a SANE will be licensed as an RN. After completing a SANE program and supervised patient encounters, the nurse will be eligible to sit for a certifying examination offered by the IAFN Forensic Nursing Certification Board. The certified SANE will receive victims of sexual assault and practice in a setting, such as emergency rooms, that is commensurate with nursing education and experience, within the scope of practice defined by professional organizations, regulatory agencies, and their institution.

Advanced Practice Forensic Nursing

Advanced practice forensic nursing incorporates expanded and specialized knowledge and skills. It is characterized by the integration and application of a range of theoretical and evidence-based knowledge acquired as a part of an advanced practice nursing graduate education. Forensic Advanced Practice Registered Nurses hold master's or doctorate degrees and are licensed, certified, and approved to practice in their roles as a clinical nurse specialist, nurse practitioner, or certified nurse midwife.

The advanced practice registered nurse or the Forensic Advanced Nursing Practice Nurse prepared as a SANE would hold a graduate degree at a minimum, or teach in a graduate curriculum in nursing with formal coursework in forensic sciences and public health or related theory, and forensic nursing applications. The graduate forensic nurse will be able to meet competencies identified in *Forensic Nursing: Scope and Standards of Practice* as well as domains located in the Core Curriculum for Forensic Advanced Practice Registered Nurses (IAFN, 2004). The practice of the forensic nurse who has a graduate nursing degree and is a SANE will differ from the generalist practice in the depth and breadth of knowledge on which nursing practice is based, and the scope of the role expectations. The graduate- or doctorate-prepared SANE would develop, promote, and implement evidence-based practice for individuals and families within systems. In addition, the graduate- or doctorate-prepared SANE would engage in research and formative and summative program evaluation in systems of care for victims and perpetrators of sexual assault and the complex health problems associated with sexual assault for individuals, families, and communities. Health promotion activities provided by the graduate- or doctorate-prepared SANE emphasize the identification and prevention of sexual assault and the resulting trauma and injury, as well as influencing systems change necessary to respond to this complex patient phenomenon in all types of communities.

In other cases, the Forensic Advanced Practice Registered Nurse collaborates with criminal justice and healthcare professionals to care for, diagnose, and treat patients impacted by injury, including follow-up care. The Forensic Advanced Practice Registered Nurse must obtain a minimum of a graduate degree in nursing with emphasis in an acknowledged specialty area (e.g., family nurse practitioner) on the prevention of trauma and the diagnosis and treatment of illnesses and responses to trauma, violence, and injury. The Forensic Advanced Practice Registered Nurse diagnoses, treats, and manages acute illness and chronic responses to injury in individuals, groups, and communities in the context of the medico-legal system. The assessment process would include obtaining health and forensic histories and conducting health and medical assessments for diagnostic purposes that include evidence collection and treatment of health outcomes. The Forensic Advanced Practice Registered Nurse prescribes medications and develops healthcare interventions within the scope of practice defined by professional organizations, regulatory agencies, and institutions. Health promotion activities of the advanced practice registered nurse and the Forensic Advanced Nursing Practice Nurse emphasize the identification and prevention of risks associated with violence, trauma, and injury in systems that respond to care of patients.

Ethics and Forensic Nursing

Based on the belief that human worth is the philosophical foundation on which forensic nursing is based, the practice of forensic nursing is consistent with IAFN's *Code of Ethics for Forensic Nurses* (2006), the *International Code of Ethics for Nurses* (ICNurses, 2006), and the *Code of Ethics for Nurses with Interpretative Statements* (ANA, 2001, 2005a)

Forensic nurses demonstrate an awareness of and adherence to regional and international laws governing their practice. Forensic nurses uphold ethical principles promoted by the nursing profession that protect the rights of, and advocate for, individuals, families, and communities in the systems that respond to them. The forensic nurse seeks evidence-based resources related to the health, safety, legal, and ethical issues for the forensic patient. Forensic nurses deliver services in a non-judgmental and non-discriminatory manner that is sensitive to diversity of the patient and the community. The forensic nurse practices with compassion and respect for the uniqueness of patients, including the moral and legal rights associated with self-determination within forensic settings and systems. Forensic nurses collaborate to address the forensic health needs of the patient, but when conflicting situations arise from previous bias and victimization, addiction, vicarious trauma, or interprofessional situations, the forensic nurse will examine the conflicts between personal and professional values, strive to preserve the patient's best interest, and preserve their professional integrity by establishing boundaries.

Nurses have a lifelong commitment to learning and maintenance of competence. This includes self-evaluation, coupled with peer review, to ensure that the forensic nursing practice is held to the highest standard. Nurses are required to have knowledge relevant to the current forensic nursing scope and standards of practice, including relevant changing issues, forensic nursing and nursing ethics, concerns, and controversies. Forensic nurses participate in the advancement of practice through administration, education, and knowledge development as well as advancing the profession through healthcare policy, professional standards, and dissemination of knowledge germane to forensic nursing practice. This may come from shared domains in nursing (such as public health, genetics and genomics) or other professions (such as medicine, public health, and forensic science). Most importantly, the forensic nurse has responsibilities to the public to respond appropriately to improve access to forensic nursing care and to bring about social change that creates a world without violence (ANA, 2001, 2005a; Canadian Nurses Association, 2002; IAFN, 2006; ICN, 2006).

Goals, Trends, and Issues in Forensic Nursing

The needs and expectations of society will shape the future of the specialty in a technologically savvy environment. Collaborating individuals, communities, organizations, and governments who support the development of the forensic nursing role will bring the forensic nurse specialist international recognition. The specialty knowledge, with acceptance and understanding of the scope and standards of practice, will continue to improve the response to patients who need forensic healthcare in interprofessional systems worldwide.

Education

Forensic nursing educational programs will continue to grow as an increasing number of accredited universities and colleges develop master's and doctorate curricula in the specialty of forensic nursing worldwide (AACN, 1998, 2006). The master's and doctorate education will reflect the expansion of the scientific evidence base of forensic nursing. Forensic nursing education will follow the trends for specialties using distance learning based on advanced technology, electronically supported simulations, and telemedicine. This trend will support access to education for and by master's and doctorate forensic nurses in remote locations worldwide and, in turn, will provide access to quality forensic nursing care to the patient populations residing in their remote communities. Future forensic nurses will assume leadership positions and create new venues for forensic nurse practice, such as entrepreneurial activities and legislative representation. Future forensic nurses will influence nursing practice because at all levels of nursing education, elements of forensic nursing content are and will continue to be threaded throughout nursing coursework.

Research

Research, as a foundation for evidence-based practice, supports the forensic nurse role. With technological advances in informatics and communication, forensic nursing research will develop at a rapid pace as clinical, educational, and administrative Forensic Advanced Practice Registered Nurses will require and produce scientific evidence in support of their growing practices. Informatics will provide the conduit for the rapid dissemination of forensic nursing research (O'Carroll & Public Health Informatics Competencies Working Group, 2002). Forensic nursing research will influence government policy, legislation, and action as the scientific base increases and graduate education, experience, and credentialing processes are realized by the forensic nursing community. It is also projected that the international interprofessional community will increasingly acknowledge the forensic nurse as a valuable interprofessional team member where healthcare and legal systems intersect.

Population Focus

Forensic nursing and public health nursing are inextricably linked both locally and in international cultures and systems, particularly in the primary, secondary, and tertiary care of intentional and unintentional injury involving individuals, families, communities, and populations. Future master's and doctorate curriculums internationally will use the graduate public health nursing competencies (QUAD Council, 2003) as a basis for forensic care of populations by nurses, an essential requirement in master's and doctorate education competencies (AACN, 2006). In addition, the population emphasis on prevention, health promotion, and program formative and summative evaluation and sustainability will help meet pressing needs in patient populations at risk for injury from intentional and unintentional violence. The population-focused approaches toward man-made or weather-related disaster and mass casualty will merge population care with intentional and unintentional injury aspects of the two disciplines—forensic nursing and public health nursing. The forensic nursing specialist will influence policy, practice, and trends when tackling issues of population-focused care related to intentional and unintentional injury prevention and intervention. As a well-educated and respected professional, the graduate forensic nurse will link public health principles and forensic science to forensic nursing practice to create a foundation for the evaluation and treatment of injury in populations worldwide.

Genetics and Genomics

Technology will provide future forensic nurses with tremendous information about patients affected by genetic healthcare problems who seek care in a forensic setting (Consensus Panel, 2006). With the integration of genetic and genomic knowledge in nursing curricula, future forensic nurses will understand the relationships between health and genetics and genomics as it relates to violence, violent behavior, and victimization. Forensic nurses will also provide services based on culture, religion, knowledge level, literacy, and preferred language in the context of the forensic healthcare presentation in the patient, whether individual, family, community, or population.

STANDARDS OF FORENSIC NURSING PRACTICE

Function of Standards

The Standards, which are comprised of the standards of practice (pages 23–34) and the standards of professional performance (pages 35–48), are authoritative statements by which nurses practicing within the role, population, and specialty governed by this document (*Forensic Nursing: Scope and Standards of Practice*) that describe the duties that they are expected to competently perform. The Standards published herein may be utilized as evidence of the legal standard of care governing nurses practicing within the role, population, and specialty governed by this document. The Standards are subject to change with the dynamics of the nursing profession and as new patterns of professional practice are developed and accepted by the nursing profession and the public. In addition, specific conditions and clinical circumstances may also affect the application of the Standards at a given time; e.g., during a natural disaster. The Standards are subject to formal, periodic review and revision.

The measurement criteria that appear below each standard are not all-inclusive and do not establish the legal standard of care. Rather, the measurement criteria are specific, measurable elements that can be used by nursing professionals to measure professional performance. Nurses practicing within this particular role, population, and specialty can identify opportunities for development and improvement by evaluating performance on these elements.

STANDARDS OF PRACTICE

STANDARD 1. ASSESSMENT
The forensic nurse collects comprehensive data pertinent to the patient's health or the situation.

Measurement Criteria:

The forensic nurse:

- Collects data in a systematic and ongoing process with a focus on identifying the medical–legal implications of those findings.

- Involves the patient, family, community, nurses and other health-care providers, interprofessional personnel, and environment, as appropriate, in collaborative holistic data collection.

- Prioritizes data collection activities based on the patient's immediate condition, anticipated needs of the patient or situation, and preservation of legal evidence.

- Uses appropriate evidence-based assessment techniques and instruments in collecting pertinent data.

- Uses analytical models and problem-solving tools in forensic nursing practice.

- Synthesizes available data, information, and knowledge relevant to the situation to identify patterns and variances.

- Documents relevant data in a retrievable format.

Additional Measurement Criteria for the Forensic Advanced Practice Registered Nurse:

The Forensic Advanced Practice Registered Nurse:

- Initiates and interprets diagnostic tests and procedures relevant to the specific area of forensic nursing practice.

STANDARD 2. DIAGNOSIS

The forensic nurse analyzes the assessment data to determine the diagnoses or issues.

Measurement Criteria:

The forensic nurse:

- Derives the diagnoses or issues based on assessment data.

- Validates the diagnoses or issues with the patient, family, and other healthcare providers when possible and appropriate.

- Documents diagnoses or issues in a manner that facilitates the determination of the expected outcomes and plan.

Additional Measurement Criteria for the Forensic Advanced Practice Registered Nurse:

The Forensic Advanced Practice Registered Nurse:

- Systematically compares and contrasts clinical findings with normal and abnormal variations and developmental events in formulating a differential diagnosis.

- Utilizes complex data and information obtained during interview, examination, diagnostic procedures, and review of medical–legal evidentiary documents in identifying diagnoses.

- Assists staff in developing and maintaining competency in the diagnostic process.

STANDARD 3. OUTCOMES IDENTIFICATION
The forensic nurse identifies expected outcomes for a plan individualized to the patient or the situation.

Measurement Criteria:

The forensic nurse:

- Involves the patient, family, other healthcare providers, and other collaborating professionals, in formulating expected outcomes when possible and appropriate.

- Derives culturally appropriate expected outcomes from the diagnoses.

- Considers associated risks, benefits, costs, current scientific evidence, medical–legal factors, and clinical expertise when formulating expected outcomes.

- Defines expected outcomes in terms of the patient, patient values, ethical considerations, environment, or situation with such considerations as associated risks, benefits and costs, and current scientific evidence.

- Includes a time estimate for attainment of expected outcomes when appropriate.

- Develops expected outcomes that provide direction for continuity of care.

- Modifies expected outcomes based on changes in the status of the patient or evaluation of the situation.

- Documents expected outcomes as measurable goals.

Additional Measurement Criteria for the Forensic Advanced Practice Registered Nurse:

The Forensic Advanced Practice Registered Nurse:

- Identifies expected outcomes that incorporate scientific evidence and are achievable through implementation of evidence-based practices.

- Identifies expected outcomes that incorporate cost and clinical effectiveness, patient satisfaction, community safety, and continuity and consistency among providers.

- Supports the use of clinical guidelines linked to positive patient outcomes.

STANDARD 4. PLANNING

The forensic nurse develops a plan that prescribes strategies and alternatives to attain expected outcomes.

Measurement Criteria:

The forensic nurse:

- Develops an individualized plan considering patient characteristics or the situation (e.g., age- and culturally appropriate, environmentally sensitive).

- Develops the plan in conjunction with the patient, family, and others, as appropriate.

- Includes strategies in the plan that address each of the identified diagnoses or issues, which may include strategies for promotion and restoration of health and prevention of illness, injury, and disease.

- Provides for continuity in the plan.

- Incorporates an implementation pathway or timeline in the plan.

- Establishes the plan priorities with the patient, family, and others as appropriate.

- Utilizes the plan to provide direction to other members of the healthcare and interprofessional team.

- Defines the plan to reflect current statutes, rules and regulations, and standards.

- Integrates current trends and research affecting care in planning.

- Considers the economic impact of the plan.

- Uses standardized language or recognized terminology to document the plan.

Additional Measurement Criteria for the Forensic Advanced Practice Registered Nurse:

The Forensic Advanced Practice Registered Nurse:

- Identifies assessment and diagnostic strategies and therapeutic interventions in the plan that reflect current evidence, including data, research, literature, and expert clinical knowledge.

- Selects or designs strategies to meet the multifaceted needs of complex patients and situations.

- Includes the synthesis of patients' values and beliefs regarding nursing and medical therapies in the plan.

Additional Measurement Criteria for the Nursing Role Specialty:

The forensic nurse in a nursing role specialty:

- Participates in the design and development of interprofessional and multi/inter-disciplinary processes to address the forensic situation or issue.

- Contributes to the development, evaluation, and continuous improvement of organizational systems that support planning.

- Supports the integration of clinical, human, medical–legal, social, and financial resources to enhance and complete decision-making.

STANDARD 5. IMPLEMENTATION
The forensic nurse implements the identified plan.

Measurement Criteria:

The forensic nurse:

- Implements the plan in a safe and timely manner.
- Documents implementation and any modifications, including changes or omissions, of the identified plan.
- Utilizes evidence-based interventions and treatments specific to the diagnosis or problem.
- Utilizes community resources and systems to implement the plan.
- Collaborates with nursing colleagues and others to implement the plan.

Additional Measurement Criteria for the Forensic Advanced Practice Registered Nurse:

The Forensic Advanced Practice Registered Nurse:

- Facilitates modification and utilization of systems and community resources to implement the plan.
- Supports collaboration with nursing colleagues and other disciplines and professions to implement the plan.
- Incorporates new knowledge and strategies to initiate change in nursing care practices if desired outcomes are not achieved.

Additional Measurement Criteria for the Nursing Role Specialty:

The forensic nurse in a nursing role specialty:

- Implements the plan using principles and concepts of project or systems management.
- Fosters organizational systems that support implementation of the plan.

STANDARD 5A: COORDINATION OF CARE
The forensic nurse coordinates care delivery.

Measurement Criteria:

The forensic nurse:

- Coordinates implementation of the plan.
- Documents the coordination of the care and the plan.

Measurement Criteria for the Forensic Advanced Practice Registered Nurse:

The Forensic Advanced Practice Registered Nurse:

- Provides leadership in the administration and coordination of interprofessional health care for integrated delivery of patient care services.
- Synthesizes data and information to prescribe necessary system and community support measures, including environmental modifications.
- Coordinates system and community resources that enhance delivery of care across continuums.

STANDARD 5B: HEALTH TEACHING AND HEALTH PROMOTION

The forensic nurse employs strategies to promote health and a safe environment.

Measurement Criteria:

The forensic nurse:

- Provides health teaching that addresses such topics as healthy lifestyles, risk-reducing behaviors, developmental needs, activities of daily living, and preventive self care.

- Uses health promotion and health teaching methods appropriate to the situation and the patient's developmental level, learning needs, readiness, ability to learn, language preference, and culture.

- Seeks opportunities for feedback and evaluation of the effectiveness of the strategies used.

Additional Measurement Criteria for the Forensic Advanced Practice Registered Nurse:

The Forensic Advanced Practice Registered Nurse:

- Synthesizes empirical evidence on risk behaviors, learning theories, behavioral change theories, motivational theories, epidemiology, and other related theories and frameworks when designing health information and patient education.

- Designs health information and patient education appropriate to the patient's developmental level, learning needs, readiness to learn, and cultural values and beliefs.

- Evaluates health information resources, such as the Internet, in the area of practice for accuracy, readability, and comprehensibility to help patients access quality health information.

STANDARD 5C: CONSULTATION

The Forensic Advanced Practice Registered Nurse and the nursing role specialist provide consultation to influence the identified plan, enhance the abilities of others, and effect change.

Measurement Criteria for the Forensic Advanced Practice Registered Nurse:

The Forensic Advanced Practice Registered Nurse:

- Synthesizes clinical data, theoretical frameworks, and evidence when providing consultation.

- Facilitates the effectiveness of a consultation by involving the patient in making decisions and negotiating role responsibilities.

- Communicates consultation recommendations that facilitate change.

Measurement Criteria for the Nursing Role Specialty

The forensic nurse in a nursing role specialty:

- Synthesizes data, information, theoretical frameworks, and evidence when providing consultation.

- Facilitates the effectiveness of a consultation by involving the stakeholders in the decision-making process.

- Communicates consultation recommendations that influence the identified plan, facilitate understanding by involved stakeholders, enhance the work of others, and effect change.

STANDARD 5D: PRESCRIPTIVE AUTHORITY AND TREATMENT
The Forensic Advanced Practice Registered Nurse uses prescriptive authority, procedures, referrals, treatments, and therapies in accordance with state and federal laws and regulations.

Measurement Criteria for the Forensic Advanced Practice Registered Nurse:

The Forensic Advanced Practice Registered Nurse:

- Prescribes evidence-based treatments, therapies, and procedures considering the patient's comprehensive healthcare needs.

- Prescribes pharmacologic agents based on a current knowledge of pharmacology and physiology.

- Prescribes specific pharmacological agents or treatments based on clinical indicators, the patient's status and needs, and the results of diagnostic and laboratory tests.

- Evaluates therapeutic and potential adverse effects of pharmacological and non-pharmacological treatments.

- Provides patients with information about intended effects and potential adverse effects of proposed prescriptive therapies.

- Provides information about costs and alternative treatments and procedures, as appropriate.

STANDARD 6. EVALUATION
The forensic nurse evaluates progress towards attainment of outcomes.

Measurement Criteria:

The forensic nurse:

- Conducts a systematic, ongoing, and criterion-based evaluation of the outcomes in relation to the structures and processes prescribed by the plan and the indicated timeline.
- Includes the patient and others involved in the care or situation in the evaluation process.
- Evaluates the effectiveness of the planned strategies in relation to patient responses and the attainment of the expected outcomes.
- Documents the results of the evaluation.
- Uses ongoing assessment data to revise the diagnoses, outcomes, the plan, and the implementation as needed.
- Disseminates the results to the patient and others involved in the care or situation, as appropriate, in accordance with state and federal laws and regulations.

Additional Measurement Criteria for the Forensic Advanced Practice Registered Nurse:

The Forensic Advanced Practice Registered Nurse:

- Evaluates the accuracy of the diagnosis and the effectiveness of the interventions in relation to the patient's attainment of expected outcomes.
- Synthesizes the results of the evaluation analyses to determine the impact of the plan on the affected patients, families, groups, communities, and institutions.
- Uses the results of the evaluation analyses to make or recommend process or structural changes including policy, procedure, or protocol documentation, as appropriate.

Continued ▶

Additional Measurement Criteria for the Nursing Role Specialty:

The forensic nurse in a nursing role specialty:

- Uses the results of the evaluation analyses to make or recommend process or structural changes including policy, procedure, or protocol documentation, as appropriate.

- Synthesizes the results of the evaluation analyses to determine the impact of the plan on the affected patients, families, groups, communities, institutions, networks, and organizations.

STANDARDS OF PROFESSIONAL PERFORMANCE

STANDARDS OF PROFESSIONAL PERFORMANCE

STANDARD 7. QUALITY OF PRACTICE
The forensic nurse systematically enhances the quality and effectiveness of forensic nursing practice.

Measurement Criteria:

The forensic nurse:

- Demonstrates quality by documenting the application of the nursing process in a responsible, accountable, and ethical manner.

- Uses the results of quality improvement activities to initiate changes in forensic nursing practice and in the healthcare delivery system.

- Uses creativity and innovation in forensic nursing practice to improve care delivery.

- Incorporates new knowledge to initiate changes in forensic nursing practice if desired outcomes are not achieved.

- Participates in quality improvement activities such as:

  - Identifying aspects of forensic nursing practice important for quality monitoring.

  - Using indicators developed to monitor quality and effectiveness of forensic nursing practice.

  - Collecting data to monitor quality and effectiveness of forensic nursing practice.

  - Analyzing quality data to identify opportunities for improving forensic nursing practice.

  - Formulating recommendations to improve forensic nursing practice or outcomes.

  - Taking action to enhance the quality of forensic nursing practice.

  - Developing, implementing, and evaluating policies, procedures, and guidelines to improve the quality of forensic nursing practice.

Continued ▶

- Participating on interprofessional teams to evaluate clinical care or health services.
- Participating in efforts to minimize costs and unnecessary duplication.
- Analyzing factors related to safety, satisfaction, effectiveness, and cost–benefit options.
- Analyzing organizational systems for barriers.
- Implementing processes to remove or decrease barriers in organizational systems.

Additional Measurement Criteria for the Forensic Advanced Practice Registered Nurse:

The Forensic Advanced Practice Registered Nurse:

- Obtains and maintains professional certification if available in the area of expertise.
- Designs quality improvement initiatives.
- Implements initiatives to evaluate the need for change.
- Evaluates the practice environment and quality of nursing care rendered in relation to existing evidence, identifying opportunities for the generation and use of research.

Additional Measurement Criteria for the Nursing Role Specialty:

The forensic nurse in a nursing role specialty:

- Obtains and maintains professional certification if available in the area of expertise.
- Designs quality improvement initiatives.
- Implements initiatives to evaluate the need for change.
- Evaluates the practice environment in relation to existing evidence, identifying opportunities for the generation and use of research.

STANDARD 8. EDUCATION
The forensic nurse attains knowledge and competency that reflect current nursing practice.

Measurement Criteria:

The forensic nurse:

- Participates in ongoing educational activities related to appropriate knowledge bases and professional issues.
- Demonstrates a commitment to lifelong learning through self-reflection and inquiry to identify learning needs.
- Seeks experiences that reflect current practice in order to maintain skills and competence in clinical practice or role performance.
- Acquires knowledge and skills appropriate to the specialty area, practice setting, role, or situation.
- Maintains professional records that provide evidence of competency and lifelong learning.
- Seeks experiences and formal and independent learning activities to maintain and develop clinical and professional skills and knowledge.

Additional Measurement Criteria for the Forensic Advanced Practice Registered Nurse:

The Forensic Advanced Practice Registered Nurse:

- Uses current healthcare research findings and other evidence to expand clinical knowledge, enhance role performance, and increase knowledge of professional issues.

Additional Measurement Criteria for the Nursing Role Specialty:

The forensic nurse in a nursing role specialty:

- Uses current research findings and other evidence to expand knowledge, enhance role performance, and increase knowledge of professional issues.

STANDARD 9. PROFESSIONAL PRACTICE EVALUATION

The forensic nurse evaluates one's own nursing practice in relation to professional practice standards and guidelines, relevant statutes, rules, and regulations.

Measurement Criteria:

The forensic nurse's practice reflects the application of knowledge of current practice standards, guidelines, statutes, rules, and regulations. The forensic nurse:

- Provides age-appropriate care in a culturally and ethnically sensitive manner.

- Engages in self-evaluation of practice on a regular basis, identifying areas of strength as well as areas in which professional development would be beneficial.

- Obtains informal feedback regarding one's own practice from patients, peers, professional colleagues, and others.

- Participates in systematic peer review as appropriate.

- Takes action to achieve goals identified during the evaluation process.

- Provides rationales for practice beliefs, decisions, and actions as part of the informal and formal evaluation processes.

Additional Measurement Criteria for the Forensic Advanced Practice Registered Nurse:

The Forensic Advanced Practice Registered Nurse:

- Engages in a formal process seeking feedback regarding one's own practice from patients, peers, professional colleagues, and others.

Additional Measurement Criteria for the Nursing Role Specialty:

The forensic nurse in a nursing role specialty:

- Engages in a formal process seeking feedback regarding role performance from individuals, professional colleagues, representatives and administrators of corporate entities, and others.

STANDARD 10. COLLEGIALITY

The forensic nurse interacts with, and contributes to the professional development of, peers and colleagues.

Measurement Criteria:

The forensic nurse:

- Shares knowledge and skills with peers and colleagues as evidenced by such activities as patient care conferences or presentations at formal or informal meetings.

- Provides peers with feedback regarding their practice or role performance.

- Interacts with peers and colleagues to enhance one's own professional nursing practice and role performance.

- Maintains compassionate and caring relationships with peers and colleagues.

- Contributes to an environment that is conducive to the education of healthcare professionals.

- Contributes to a supportive and healthy work environment.

Additional Measurement Criteria for the Forensic Advanced Practice Registered Nurse:

The Forensic Advanced Practice Registered Nurse:

- Models expert practice to other nurses, interprofessional team members, and healthcare consumers.

- Mentors other registered nurses and colleagues as appropriate.

- Participates with teams that contribute to role development and advanced nursing practice and health care.

Additional Measurement Criteria for the Nursing Role Specialty:

The forensic nurse in a nursing role specialty:

- Participates on interprofessional and nursing teams that contribute to role development and, directly or indirectly, advance nursing practice and health services.

- Mentors other registered nurses and colleagues as appropriate.

STANDARD 11. COLLABORATION
The forensic nurse collaborates with patient, family, and others in the conduct of nursing practice.

Measurement Criteria:

The forensic nurse:

- Communicates with patient, family, and healthcare providers regarding patient care and the nurse's role in the provision of that care.

- Collaborates in creating a documented plan focused on outcomes and decisions related to care and delivery of services that indicates communication with patients, families, and others.

- Partners with others to effect change and generate positive outcomes through knowledge of the patient or situation.

- Documents referrals, including provisions for continuity of care.

Additional Measurement Criteria for the Forensic Advanced Practice Registered Nurse:

The Forensic Advanced Practice Registered Nurse:

- Partners with other disciplines to enhance patient care through interprofessional activities, such as education, consultation, management, technological development, or research opportunities.

- Facilitates an interprofessional process with other members of the healthcare team.

- Documents plan-of-care communications, rationales for plan-of-care changes, and collaborative discussions to improve patient care.

Additional Measurement Criteria for Nursing Role Specialty:

The forensic nurse in a nursing role specialty:

- Partners with others to enhance health care, and ultimately patient care, through interprofessional activities such as education, consultation, management, technological development, or research opportunities.

- Documents plans, communications, rationales for plan changes, and collaborative discussions.

STANDARD 12. ETHICS
The forensic nurse integrates ethical provisions in all areas of practice.

Measurement Criteria:

The forensic nurse:

- Uses *Code of Ethics for Nurses with Interpretive Statements* (ANA, 2001) and *Forensic Nurse's Code of Ethics* (IAFN, 2006) to guide practice.

- Delivers care in a manner that protects patient autonomy, dignity, and rights.

- Maintains patient confidentiality within legal and regulatory parameters.

- Serves as a patient advocate assisting patients in developing skills for self-advocacy and empowerment.

- Maintains a therapeutic and professional patient–nurse relationship within appropriate professional role boundaries.

- Demonstrates a commitment to practicing self-care, managing stress, and connecting with self and others.

- Contributes to resolving ethical issues of patients, colleagues, or systems as evidenced in such activities as participating on ethics committees.

- Reports illegal, incompetent, or impaired practices.

Additional Measurement Criteria for the Forensic Advanced Practice Registered Nurse:

The Forensic Advanced Practice Registered Nurse:

- Informs the patient of the risks, benefits, and outcomes of health-care regimens.

- Participates in interprofessional and nursing teams that address ethical risks, benefits, and outcomes for patients.

Continued ▶

Additional Measurement Criteria for the Nursing Role Specialty:

The forensic nurse in a nursing role specialty:

- Participates on interprofessional teams that address ethical risks, benefits, and outcomes.

- Informs administrators or others of the risks, benefits, and outcomes of programs and decisions that affect healthcare delivery.

STANDARD 13. RESEARCH
The forensic nurse integrates research findings into practice.

Measurement Criteria:

The forensic nurse:

- Utilizes the best available evidence, including research findings, to guide practice decisions.

- Actively participates in research activities at various levels appropriate to the nurse's level of education and position. Such activities may include:

  - Identifying clinical problems specific to nursing research (patient care and forensic nursing practice).

  - Participating in data collection (such as, but not limited to surveys, pilot projects, formal studies).

  - Participating in formal committees or programs.

  - Sharing research and findings with peers and others.

  - Conducting research.

  - Critically analyzing and interpreting research for application to practice.

  - Using research findings in the development of policies, procedures, and standards of practice in patient care.

  - Incorporating research as a basis for learning.

Additional Measurement Criteria for the Forensic Advanced Practice Registered Nurse:

The Forensic Advanced Practice Registered Nurse:

- Contributes to nursing knowledge by conducting or synthesizing research that discovers, examines, and evaluates knowledge, theories, criteria, and creative approaches to improve healthcare practice.

- Formally disseminates research findings through activities such as presentations, publications, consultation, and journal clubs.

Continued ▶

Additional Measurement Criteria for the Nursing Role Specialty:

The forensic nurse in a nursing role specialty:

- Contributes to nursing knowledge by conducting or synthesizing research that discovers, examines, and evaluates knowledge, theories, criteria, and creative approaches to improve health care.
- Formally disseminates research findings through activities such as presentations, publications, consultation, and journal clubs.

STANDARD 14. RESOURCE UTILIZATION

The forensic nurse considers factors related to safety, effectiveness, cost, and impact on practice in the planning and delivery of nursing services.

Measurement Criteria:

The forensic nurse:

- Evaluates factors such as safety, effectiveness, availability, cost–benefits, efficiencies, and impact on practice, when choosing among practice options that would result in the same expected outcome.

- Assists the patient and family in identifying and securing appropriate and available services to address health-related needs.

- Assigns or delegates tasks, based on the needs and condition of the patient, potential for harm, stability of the patient's condition, complexity of the task, and predictability of the outcome.

- Assists the patient and family in becoming informed consumers about the options, costs, risks, and benefits of treatment and care.

Additional Measurement Criteria for the Forensic Advanced Practice Registered Nurse:

The Forensic Advanced Practice Registered Nurse:

- Utilizes organizational and community resources to formulate interprofessional plans of care.

- Develops innovative solutions for patient care problems that address effective resource utilization and maintenance of quality.

- Develops strategies to evaluate cost-effectiveness associated with nursing practice.

Additional Measurement Criteria for the Nursing Role Specialty:

The forensic nurse in a nursing role specialty:

- Develops innovative solutions and applies strategies to obtain appropriate resources for nursing initiatives.

Continued ▶

- Secures organizational resources to ensure a work environment conducive to completing the identified plan and outcomes.

- Develops formative and summative evaluation methods to measure safety and effectiveness for interventions and outcomes.

- Promotes activities that assist others, as appropriate, in becoming informed about costs, risks, and benefits of care or of the plan and solution.

STANDARD 15. LEADERSHIP

The forensic nurse provides leadership in the professional practice setting and the profession.

Measurement Criteria:

The forensic nurse:

- Engages in teamwork as a team player and a team builder.

- Works to create and maintain healthy work environments in local, regional, national, or international communities.

- Displays the ability to define a clear vision, the associated goals, and a plan to implement and measure progress.

- Demonstrates a commitment to continuous, lifelong learning for self and others.

- Teaches others to succeed by mentoring and other strategies.

- Exhibits creativity and flexibility through times of change.

- Demonstrates energy, excitement, and a passion for quality work.

- Willingly accepts mistakes by self and others, thereby creating a culture in which risk-taking is not only safe, but expected.

- Inspires loyalty by valuing people as the most precious asset in an organization.

- Directs the coordination of care across settings and among care-givers, including oversight of licensed and unlicensed personnel in any assigned or delegated tasks.

- Serves in key roles in the work setting by assuming leadership positions on committees, councils, and administrative teams.

- Promotes advancement of the profession through active participation in professional organizations.

Continued ▶

Additional Measurement Criteria for the Forensic Advanced Practice Registered Nurse:

The Forensic Advanced Practice Registered Nurse:

- Works to influence decision-making bodies to improve patient care.

- Provides direction to enhance the effectiveness of the healthcare and interprofessional team.

- Initiates and revises protocols or guidelines to reflect evidence-based practice, to reflect accepted changes in care management, or to address emerging problems.

- Promotes communication of information and advancement of the profession through writing, publishing, and presentations for inter-professional or lay audiences.

- Designs innovations to effect change in practice and improves health outcomes.

Additional Measurement Criteria for the Nursing Role Specialty:

The forensic nurse in a nursing role specialty:

- Works to influence decision-making bodies to improve patient care, health services, and policies.

- Promotes communication of information and advancement of the profession through writing, publishing, and presentations for professional or lay audiences.

- Designs innovations to effect change in practice and outcomes.

- Provides evidence-based direction and leadership to enhance the effectiveness of interprofessional teams.

GLOSSARY

Assessment. A systematic, dynamic process by which the registered nurse collects and analyzes data (ANA, 2004). In forensic settings: (1) the RN interacts with the patient, family, groups, communities, populations, healthcare providers, public health and law enforcement agencies, and medical and judicial systems; (2) may include these dimensions: physical, psychological, sociocultural, spiritual, cognitive, functional abilities, developmental, economic, cultural, and lifestyle.

Certification. Tangible recognition of professional achievement in a defined functional or clinical area of nursing (American Board of Nursing Specialties, 2005, n.d.).

Continuity of care. A process that involves patients, families, significant others, and interprofessional team members in the determination of a coordinated plan of care. This process facilitates the patient's transition between settings, healthcare providers, and interprofessional agencies, and is based on changing needs and available resources in the community.

Diagnosis. A judgment about the response to actual or potential health conditions or needs; the diagnosis provides the basis for determination of a plan of services to achieve expected outcomes; registered nurses in forensic settings utilize nursing or medical diagnoses depending on educational and clinical preparation and legal authority.

Environment. The atmosphere, milieu, or condition in which an individual lives, works, or plays (ANA, 2004).

Evaluation. The process of determining the progress toward the attainment of expected outcomes; outcomes include the effectiveness of care, when addressing one's practice (ANA, 2004).

Evidence-based practice. A process founded on the collection, interpretation, and integration of valid, important, and applicable patient-reported, clinician-observed, and research-derived evidence. The best available evidence, moderated by patient circumstances and preferences, is applied to improve the quality of clinical judgments (ANA, 2004).

Family. Family of origin or significant others as identified by the patient (ANA, 2004).

Forensic. Pertaining to law; for the purposes of this document, relating to the use of science or technology in the investigation and establishment of facts or evidence (Merriam-Webster's 2008).

Forensic Advanced Practice Registered Nurse. A licensed registered nurse who has completed graduate or doctoral education with a specialization or emphasis in forensic nursing, and holds Advanced Practice Registered Nurse (APRN) credentials as a Clinical Nurse Specialist, Certified Nurse-Midwife, or Nurse Practitioner.

Forensic nursing. "The practice of nursing globally where health and legal systems intersect" (IAFN, 2008).

Formative evaluation. The structured development of processes or programs including the goals, outcomes, and output identification (Weiss, 1998). In the forensic nursing process and programs this can inlcude setting program goals, objectives, developing measurement tools, and creating action plans that identify outcomes and outputs of the process or program.

Guidelines. Systematically developed statements that describe recommended actions based on available scientific evidence and expert opinion. Clinical guidelines describe a process of patient care management that has the potential of improving the quality of clinical and consumer decision making (ANA, 2004).

Holistic. Based on an understanding that the patient is an interconnected unity and that physical, mental, social, and spiritual factors need to be included in interventions (ANA, 2004).

Illness. The subjective experience of discomfort (ANA, 2004).

Implementation. Activities such as teaching, monitoring, providing, counseling, delegating, and coordinating (ANA, 2004) and , in forensic settings, administration.

Injury. Trauma; any damage or harm done to or suffered by a person or thing that involves the bio-psycho-social, spiritual, or financial state of an individual, family, community, or system for which legal redress may be available.

Interprofessional. Founded on engagement between professions, such as prosecutors, law enforcement officers, nurses, judges, and police officers; or between physicians and nurses. (See also *Multidisciplinary*.)

Legal. Pertaining to the law; used for the purposes of this document as a broad term to describe criminal and civil justice systems and investigative disciplines.

Multidisciplinary. Reliance on each team member or discipline contributing discipline-specific skills (ANA, 2004); in forensic nursing, usually means *interprofessional*.

Nursing. Protection, promotion, and optimization of health and abilities, prevention of illness and injury, alleviation of suffering through the diagnosis and treatment of human response, and advocacy in the care of individuals, families, communities, and populations (ANA, 2003, 2004).

Offender. One who commits, executes, or performs a criminal act of any kind and whose profiles and treatment modalities are integral to forensic nursing practice. (See also *Perpetrator*.)

Outcomes. Measurable, expected goals.

Outputs. Measurable, tangible products.

Patient. The recipient of forensic nursing practice, whether an individual, family, community, or population. The recipient may also be called client, resident, group, or system (ANA, 2004).

- When the patient is an *individual*, the focus is the health state, problems, or needs of a single person.

- When the patient is a *family* or a *group*, the focus is on the health state of that unit as a whole or the reciprocal effects of any individual's health state on any other members of the unit.

- When the patient is a *community* or *population*, the focus is on personal and environmental health and the health risks of the community or entire population.

Peer review. A collegial, systematic, and periodic process by which registered nurses are held accountable for their practice and that fosters refinement of their knowledge, skills, and decision-making at all levels in all areas of work, such as in their nursing practice (ANA, 2004).

Perpetrator. One who commits, executes, or performs a criminal act of any kind and whose profiles and treatment modalities are integral to forensic nursing practice. (See also *Offender.*)

Plan. A comprehensive outline of the steps to be completed to attain expected outcomes (ANA, 2004). May include any or all of intervention, delegation, or coordination. Within the plan of services, the patient, significant other, agency, service organization, law enforcement agency, judicial system, or healthcare provider may be designated to implement interventions.

Plan of action. Comprehensive outline of steps to deliver services in order to attain expected outcomes and outputs.

Providers. Individuals, service organizations, agencies, and professionals with special expertise who provide services or assistance to patients.

Quality of care. The degree to which health services for patients, families, groups, communities, or populations increase the likelihood of desired outcomes and are consistent with current professional knowledge (ANA, 2004).

Scope of practice. An authoritative statement enunciated and promulgated by the profession that defines its practice, service, or education.

Significant other. Individual who is an intimate of and significant to the patient.

Standard. An authoritative statement, defined and promoted by the profession, by which the quality of practice, service, or education can be evaluated (ANA, 2004).

Standards of practice. Authoritative statements that describe a competent level of service in the profession, including assessment, diagnosis, outcomes identification, planning, implementation, and evaluation.

Standards of professional performance. Authoritative statements that describe a competent level of behavior in the profession, including quality of practice, professional practice evaluation, education, collegiality, collaboration, ethics, research, resource utilization, and leadership.

Summative evaluation. Those evaluative processes that result in an outcome or product (Weiss, 1998). Forensic nurses participate in continuous quality improvement utilizing the foundational processes identified in a summative evaluation.

System. An assemblage of related elements that compose a unified whole, such as the legal and health systems, whose intersections provide the definitive context for forensic nursing, as well as the major systems in which forensic nurses practice:

- Healthcare (hospitals, surgery centers, community clinics)
- Investigative (medical examiner, law enforcement offices)
- Criminal Justice (district attorney, public defender offices),
- Correctional (jails, prisons, and detention centers)
- Government (military, local, state, provincial, and federal agencies)

Trauma. Injury which can be physical, psychological, emotional, spiritual, financial, or social; it can include loss of trust, safety, or security. Trauma is preventable and outcomes of trauma may be permanent or temporary. Trauma is amenable to independent or collaborative nursing intervention.

Victim. One who is acted upon and usually adversely affected by an outside incident. In forensic nursing, the victim may be the patient, the decedent, the perpetrator, the family, significant others, the suspect, the accused or falsely accused, the community, a population, a system, or the public in general.

REFERENCES

All URLs were retrieved April 13, 2009.

American Association of Colleges of Nursing (AACN). (1991). *Position statement: Physical violence against women.* Washington, DC: AACN.

American Association of Colleges of Nursing (AACN). (1998). *Essentials of baccalaureate education for professional nursing practice.* Washington, DC: AACN.

American Association of Colleges of Nursing (AACN). (2006). *The essentials of doctoral education for advanced nursing practice.* Washington, DC: AACN.

American Board of Nursing Specialties. (2005). *A position statement on the value of specialty nursing certification.* http://nursingcertification.org/pdf/value_certification.pdf.

American Board of Nursing Specialties. (n.d.). *Accreditation standards.* http://nursingcertification.org/pdf/ac_standards_short.pdf.

American Nurses Association (ANA). (2001). *Code of ethics for nurses with interpretive statements.* Silver Spring, MD: American Nurses Publishing.

American Nurses Association (ANA). (2003). *Nursing's social policy statement.* Washington, DC: Nursesbooks.org.

American Nurses Association (ANA). (2004). *Nursing: Scope and standards of practice.* Washington, DC: Nursesbooks.org.

American Nurses Association (ANA). (2005). *Recognition of a nursing specialty, approval of a specialty nursing scope of practice statement, and acknowledgment of specialty nursing standards of practice.* Paper presented at the Congress on Nursing Practice and Economics, Washington, DC.

American Nurses Association (ANA) & International Association of Forensic Nurses (IAFN). (1997). *Forensic nursing scope and standards of practice.* Washington, DC: ANA.

Burgess, A. W., Berger, A. D., & Boersma, R. R. (2004). Forensic nursing: Investigating the career potential in this emerging graduate specialty. *American Journal of Nursing, 104*(3), 58–64.

Canadian Nurses Association (CNA). (2002). *Code of ethics for registered nurses.* http://www.cna-aiic.ca/cna/documents/pdf/publications/CodeofEthics2002_e.pdf.

Canadian Nurses Association (CNA). (2007). *Framework for the practice of registered nurses in Canada.* http://www.cna-aiic.ca/CNA/documents/pdf/publications/RN_Framework_Practice_2007_e.pdf.

Canadian Nurses Association (CNA). (2008). *Advanced nursing practice: A national framework.* Ottawa, ON: Canadian Nurses Association.

Canadian Nurses Association (CNA) & Canadian Federation of Nurses Unions (CFNU). (2006). *Joint position statement. Practice environments: Maximizing client, nurse, and system outcomes.* http://www.cna-aiic.ca/CNA/documents/pdf/publications/PS88-Practice-Environments-e.pdf.

Consensus Panel on Genetic/Genomic Nursing Competencies. (2006). *Essential nursing competencies and curricula guidelines for genetics and genomics.* Silver Spring, MD: American Nurses Association.

International Association of Forensic Nurses (IAFN). (2004). *Core competencies for advanced practice forensic nursing.* http://www.forensicnurse.org/associations/8556/files/APN%20Core%20Curriculum%20Document.pdf.

International Association of Forensic Nurses (IAFN). (2006). *IAFN vision of ethical practice.* http://www.iafn.org/displaycommon.cfm?an=1&subarticlenbr=56.

International Association of Forensic Nurses (IAFN). (2008). *History of forensic nursing.* http://www.forensicnurse.org/associations/8556/files/IAFN%20Presentation.ppt#283,4,history.

International Council of Nurses (ICN). (2004). *Position statement: Scope of nursing practice.* http://www.icn.ch/psscope.htm.

International Council of Nurses (ICN). (2006). *ICN code of ethics for nurses.* Geneva: International Council of Nurses.

Koop, C. Everett. (1986). *Public health and private ethics.* http://profiles .nlm.nih.gov/QQ/B/B/F/W/_/qqbbfw.pdf.

Ledray, L. E. (1999). *SANE development and operations guide.* http:// www.ojp.usdoj.gov/ovc/publications/infores/sane/saneguide.pdf.

Lynch, V. A. (1990). *Clinical forensic nursing: A descriptive study in role development.* Unpublished thesis. Arlington, TX: University of Texas.

Mason, T., & Mercer, D. (1996). Forensic psychiatric nursing: Visions of social control. *Australian and New Zealand Journal of Mental Health Nursing, 5,* 153–162.

Merriam-Webster's collegiate dictionary, 11th ed. (2008). Springfield, MA: Merriam-Webster, Inc.

O'Carroll, P. W., & Public Health Informatics Competencies Working Group. (2002). *Informatics competencies for public health professionals.* Seattle: Northwest Center for Public Health Practice, University of Washington School of Public Health and Community Medicine.

QUAD Council. (2003). *Public Health Nursing Competencies* http:// www.sphtc.org/phn_competencies_final_comb.pdf.

Schober, M., & Affara, F. A. (2006). *International Council of Nurses: Advanced nursing practice.* Malden, MA: Blackwell Publishing.

Sheridan, D. J. (2004). Legal and forensic nursing responses to family violence. In J. Humphreys & J. C. Campbell (Eds.), *Family violence and nursing practice* (pp. 385–406). Philadelphia: Lippincott, Williams & Wilkins.

Shives, L. R. (2008). *Basic concepts of psychiatric mental health nursing* (7th ed.). Philadelphia: Lippincott, Williams, and Wilkins.

Speck, P. M. (2000). *Things you didn't learn in nursing school: Forensic nursing principles - WHEEL*. Paper presented to the Emergency Nurses Association, Chicago.

Speck, P. M., & Peters, S. (1999). Forensic nursing: Where law and nursing intersect. *Advance for Nurse Practitioners, 11*(10).

National Nursing and Nursing Education Taskforce (N³ET). (2006). *A national specialisation framework for nursing and midwifery*. Melbourne, Australia: Health Workforce Australia. http://www.nhwt.gov.au/documents/N3ET/recsp_framework.pdf

United Nations. (1948). *Universal declaration of human rights, General Assembly resolution 217 A (III)*. http://www.un.org/Overview/rights.html.

Weiss, C. H. (1998). *Evaluation* (2nd ed.). Upper Saddle River, NJ: Prentice Hall.

Appendix A
Scope and Standards of Forensic Nursing
(1997)

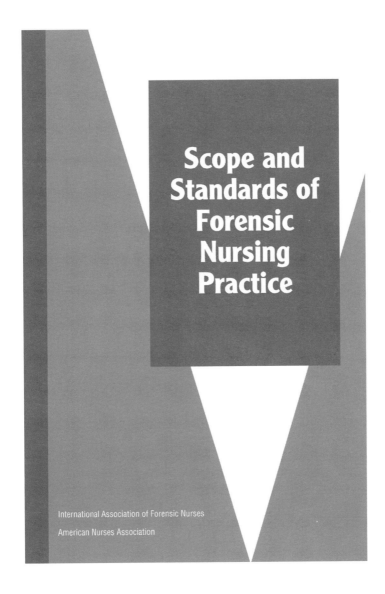

Scope and
Standards of
Forensic
Nursing
Practice

International Association of Forensic Nurses

American Nurses Association

SCOPE and STANDARDS
of Forensic
Nursing Practice

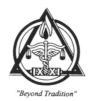

"Beyond Tradition"

INTERNATIONAL ASSOCIATION OF FORENSIC NURSES

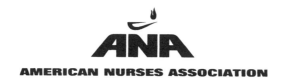

AMERICAN NURSES ASSOCIATION

This appendix is not current and is of historical significance only.

Library of Congress Cataloging-in-Publication Data

International Association of Forensic Nurses.
     Scope and standards of forensic nursing practice / International
Association of Forensic Nurses, American Nurses Association.
          p.   cm.
     Edited by Joette McHugh and Debbie Leake.
     Includes bibliographical references.
     1. Forensic nursing—Standards.   I. McHugh, Joette.   II. Leake,
Debbie.   III. American Nurses Association.   IV. Title
     [DNLM: 1. Specialties, Nursing—standards.   2. Forensic Medicine.
WY   150   I592s   1997]
RA1155.I57   1997
614' .1— DC21
DNLM/DLC
for Library of Congress   97-41343
                                                                        CIP

Published by
American Nurses Publishing
600 Maryland Ave., SW
Suite 100 West
Washington, DC 20024

First printing Dec. 1997. Second printing Apr. 1998. Third printing Feb. 1999.
Fourth printing May 2003. Fifth Printing Feb. 2004.

ST-4   .5 M   2/04R

ACKNOWLEDGMENTS

The International Association of Forensic Nurses acknowledges the contributions of those members of its Standards Committee of 1993 through 1997, who assisted in the development of the Standards and Scope of Forensic Nursing Practice, as well as others who participated in the completion of this document.

Editors:

Joette McHugh, RN
Debbie Leake, RN

Chairs of Task Force:

Suzanne L. Brown, BSN, RN, CEN
Joette McHugh, RN
Debbie Leake, RN

Contributors:

Janet Barber, MS, RN, CEN
Faye Battiste-Otto, RN
Ann W. Burgess, DNSc, RN
Robert M. Crane, BSN, RN
Patricia A.Crane, MSN, RN, NP
Marion Cumming, RN, BCFE
Catherine A. Dougherty, MA, RN
Kim Eggleston, MSN, RN
Jamie Ferrell, BSN, RN
Sheryl B. Gordon, MSN, RN
Virginia A. Lynch, MSN, RN, FAAFS
Sheila MacDonald, BSN, RN
Patty C. Seneski, RN
Diana Schunn, BSN, RN

DEDICATION

*To forensic nurses everywhere whose
commitment to going
"beyond tradition"
provides vital intervention to victims of
violent crime and
promotes the science of forensic nursing
as they prepare for health care in the 21st century.*

PREFACE

Introduction

Forensic nursing is a unique example of the innovative expansion of the role nurses will fill in the health service delivery system in the twenty-first century. Although forensic nursing is a new concept in the arena of nursing, it has been a respected practice in the scientific investigation of death for many years. It also has been recognized as a significant resource in forensic psychiatric practice and in the treatment of incarcerated patients. Today, in a precedent-setting move, the application of forensic science to the investigation of trauma in hospital emergency departments has created support for victims of violent crime. The victim can be the client, the family, the significant other, the alleged perpetrator, and the public in general. Indeed, as these needs are identified and filled by nurses, the formal recognition of forensic nursing as a discrete discipline was accomplished at the 1991 Annual Meeting of the American Academy of Forensic Sciences (February 1991, Anaheim, California). This vital link in policy for the treatment of victims of catastrophic death and near-death is a multidisciplinary issue, concerning sociologists, psychologists, social workers, political scientists, physicians, nurses, attorneys, judges and other forensic officials, advocates and activists, as well as other criminal justice system practitioners.

What is Forensic Nursing?

Forensic nursing is the application of forensic science combined with the bio-psychological education of the registered nurse, in the scientific investigation, evidence collection and preservation, analysis, prevention and treatment of trauma and/or death related medical-legal issues. The forensic nurse functions as a staff nurse, nurse scientist, nurse investigator, or as an independent consulting nurse specialist to public and/or private operatives and/or individuals in the medical-legal investigation of injury and/or death of victims of violence, criminal activity, and traumatic accidents. The forensic nurse provides direct and indirect services to individual clients, consultation services to nursing, medical and law-related agencies, as well as providing expert court testimony in areas encompassing evidence collection, preservation and analysis, questioned death investigation processes, adequacy of services delivered, and specialized diagnoses of specific conditions related to forensic nursing practice.

The focus of forensic nursing is clearly defined and represents a unique body of knowledge not found in any other specialty of nursing, forensic science or law enforcement. The forensic nurse is prepared through a synthesis of education and experience in each of these knowledge bases. This specialized education develops a clinician qualified to respond to the challenge health care faces in the protection of the legal, civil, and human rights of victims and perpetrators of violent crimes.

Forensic nursing is formally organized and is represented by a nursing specialty association. The International Association of Forensic Nurses was established in Minneapolis, Minnesota on August 12, 1992. The mission statement of the IAFN represents the concept of nurses willing to devote their energy and resources to develop a role in nursing that can have a great impact on the future of both forensic science and health care professions.

The forensic nurse is a vital component in clinical forensic practice. It is the nurse who most frequently is the first to see the patient (often the first to identify the patient as a crime victim), comes in contact with the evidence, records the medical-legal (forensic) documentation that will be used in a court of law, and contacts the grieving family. Legislation providing registered nurses the legal authority to pronounce death is being implemented in several states, in addition to the vast number of nurses being required to provide expert witness testimony in courts of law. These are prime examples of the forensic nurse as a vital component in forensic nursing practice.

Forensic nursing is further defined in the "Scope of Practice for Forensic Nurses," which was adopted by the International Association of Forensic Nurses. This scope of nursing practice was developed by the IAFN to ensure safe, competent, and ethical forensic nursing practice by those practicing within the field. It does so by providing direction to health care providers, attorneys, educators, researchers and administrators, as well as informing other health care professionals, legislators, law enforcement agencies, judicial systems, and the public about the participation in and contributions to health care by forensic nurses.

The status of our efforts to bring the application of forensic science into nursing practice remains in its embryonic stage. Only through educational programs and with the support of the American Nurses Association (ANA) will forensic nursing be viewed as an accepted and credible contributor to broadening the definition of advanced practice in the professional development of nursing.

CONTENTS

SCOPES OF FORENSIC NURSING PRACTICE

Introduction

Through needs assessment and subsequent recognition of forensic nursing as a distinct discipline, The International Association of Forensic Nurses (IAFN), as the professional association for the specialty of forensic nursing, is accountable to define and establish the scope of forensic nursing practice. The mandate of the IAFN is to ensure that safe, competent and ethical nursing care be provided to society by setting and maintaining professional standards of practice and practicing and communicating their profession according to those standards within the nursing profession and to the public. Forensic nurses are registered nurses and as such, are expected to practice in a manner consistent with the nurse practice acts set by respective State Boards of Nursing.

As a self-governing profession, nursing is responsible to define the scope of nursing practice for registered nurses. The IAFN recognizes the role of the American Nurses Association (ANA) in defining the scope of nursing practice for the nursing profession as a whole and the IAFN supports the ANA's *Nursing's Social Policy Statement*. This statement ascribes specialty nursing organizations with defining their individual scope of practice and delineating the characteristics within their unique specialty area. In using *Nursing's Social Policy Statement* as the framework for the scope of forensic nursing practice, the elements of core, dimensions, boundaries and intersections have been articulated.

Definitions

The *core* of forensic nursing specifies the definitions, roles, behaviors and processes inherent in forensic nursing practice.

The *boundaries* of forensic nursing are described as both internal and external with sufficient flexibility and resilience to change in response to societal needs and demands.

The *intersections* describe the interface of forensic nursing with other professional groups through its unique knowledge, environment, and focus.

The Speciality of Forensic Nursing

Just as the profession of nursing is diverse, so too is the specialty of forensic nursing. Most specialty nursing organizations are identified by their focus in one of the following:

- specific body system
- specific disease group
- specific age group
- specific patient/client population

Forensic nursing encompasses all of these specifications and includes the provision of care that focuses on the forensic aspects of health care combined with the bio-psychosocial education of the registered nurse in the scientific investigation and treatment of trauma and/or death of victims and perpetrators of violence, criminal activity, and traumatic accidents. The forensic nurse provides direct services to nursing, medical and/or law-related agencies, as well as providing consultation and expert testimony in areas related to questioned investigative processes, adequacy of services delivered, and specialized diagnoses of specific conditions as related to forensic nursing and/or pathology. The focus of forensic nursing is clearly defined as vital intervention by health care in advocacy and ministration to victims of violent crime, who can be the survivors, the deceased, and the families of both.

Core

The practice of a forensic nurse signifies the application of a unique dimension of nursing science to a public and/or legal community. Registered nurses within the specialty of forensic nursing can include those practicing within the arenas of:

- Forensic Nursing Sexual Assault Examiners
- Forensic Nursing Educators/Consultants
- Nurse Coroners
- Death Investigators
- Legal Nurse Consultants

- Nurse Attorneys

- Correctional Nurses

- Clinical Nursing Specialists, including those specializing in Trauma, Transplant and Critical Care Nursing

- Forensic Pediatric Nurses

- Forensic Gerontology Nurses

- Forensic Psychiatric Nurses

Forensic nursing is a unique practice of the expansive role registered nurses fill in the delivery of health care and is independent and collaborative in nature. Forensic nursing includes the delivery of care to consumers through education, research and consultation.

Forensic nurses practice within various settings whenever and wherever a medical-legal interest and forensic issues interact. This practice can occur in hospital settings; pre-hospital settings; clinics; legal arenas; businesses; educational, industrial and correctional institutes as well as other health care environments.

Dimensions

Forensic nursing is multi-dimensional and includes the responsibilities, functions, roles and skills that involve a specific body of knowledge. Characteristics unique to forensic nursing practice may include but are not limited to:

- Assessment, diagnosis, identification, planning, implementation of interventions and human responses to individuals of all ages, including but not limited to victims of sexual assault, physical assault, homicide, child abuse and spousal abuse

- Identifying injuries and deaths with forensic implications

- Collecting evidential material required by law enforcement or medical examiners

- The scientific investigation of death

- Provisions of care in uncontrolled or unpredictable environments and providing continuity of care from the emergency department to the court of law

- Crisis intervention for unique patient populations

- Expert witness testimony

- Recording the medical-legal documentation to be used in a court of law

- Interacting with grieving families

- Thoroughly reviewing and analyzing medical records

- Consulting with other agencies whenever forensic interests interact

Boundaries

The scope of forensic nursing practice is bound both externally and internally. The external boundaries include legislation and regulations, societal demands for expedient quality forensic care, economic climate and health care delivery trends. Individual State Statutes and Nurse Practice Acts are examples of legal boundaries used to provide the basis for interpreting safe practice. Additionally, rules and regulations that evolve from these acts may be used as guidelines by state boards of nursing to issue licenses and ensure public safety.

The internal boundaries include those forces that fall within the practice of professional nursing. Specific internal boundaries include the ANA guidelines for practice such as the *Nursing's Social Policy Statement* and *Standards of Clinical Practice*. Boundaries are dynamic rather than rigid. Changes within the external boundaries may be the paradigm to necessitate change to the internal boundaries.

Intersections

The practice of forensic nursing intersects with a variety of professional and governmental groups outside the domain of nursing such as law enforcement agencies, prosecuting and defense attorneys, forensic pathologists, clinical physicians, and forensic scientists. Forensic nursing also intersects with professional groups within the domain of nursing such as the American Nurses Association and other specialty nursing organizations. At these intersections, forensic nurses collaborate with other professionals toward a common goal of improving forensic collection, analysis, and health care through education, administration, consultation and collaboration in practice, research, and policy decisions by communicating, networking and sharing resources, information, research, technology, and expertise.

Summary

The depth and breadth of the scope of clinical forensic nursing practice places forensic nurses in a position to contribute significantly to health care. In this document, forensic nursing is compelled to provide direction to health care providers, educators, attorneys, researchers and administrators, as well as other health professionals, legislators, and the public in general.

Evolving professional and societal demands have necessitated a statement clarifying the scope of practice of forensic nursing practice. Given rapid changes in health care trends and technologies, this document is intended to be futuristic, allowing flexibility in response to emerging issues and practices of forensic nursing.

STANDARDS OF FORENSIC NURSING PRACTICE

Role of Standards

Standards are authoritative statements by which the nursing profession, and thus forensic nursing, describe the responsibilities for which its professionals are accountable. Consequently, standards reflect the values and priorities of the profession of forensic nursing. Standards will provide direction for professional forensic nursing practice and a framework for the evaluation of its practice. Written in measurable terms, standards also define the forensic nursing profession's accountability to the public and the outcomes for which forensic nurses are responsible.

These standards are intended for the nurse practicing within the area of forensic nursing. The forensic nurse possesses conceptual knowledge and skills gained through a specific body of knowledge including education, clinical experience, and professional development. Forensic nurses practice their science and art in a variety of settings with clients across a life span, and are sensitive to the special needs of clients from diverse cultures.

Development of Standards

Standards of professional nursing practice may pertain to general or specialty practice. Both the International Association of Forensic Nurses and the American Nurses Association have a responsibility to its membership and the public it serves, to develop standards of practice.

The development of the "Standards of Practice for Forensic Nurses" has a vital role in recognizing that forensic nursing is a unique field of nursing practiced by many nurses with diverse backgrounds. This publication has been developed in collaboration with the ANA *Standards of Clinical Practice* and describes a competent level of forensic nursing practice and professional performance common to all forensic nurses engaged in their respective practices.

Organizing Principles of the Standards of Practice for Forensic Nurses

The Scope and Standards of Forensic Nursing Practice applies to the services provided to all clients. "Clients" may include an individual, family, group or community for whom the forensic nurse provides specified services as sanctioned by nurse practice acts. These services are provided in the context of disease or injury prevention, intervention, investigation, health promotion, health restoration, maintenance, criminal investigation, evidence collection, or death investigation. The cultural, racial and ethnic diversity of the client and community must always be taken into consideration when providing forensic nursing services.

The Scope and Standards of Forensic Nursing Practice applies to all registered nurses engaged in forensic nursing practice. These standards further define the responsibilities of forensic nurses engaged in their practice who function at advanced levels of clinical practice as determined by those nursing specialties and appropriate groups within ANA.

The ANA *Standards of Clinical Nursing Practice* are the basic standards which apply to all nurses. The IAFN has utilized the *Standards of Clinical Nursing Practice* to develop specific criteria for defining expectations within the parameters of forensic nursing.

The Scope and Standards of Forensic Nursing Practice consist of "Standards of Care" and "Standards of Professional Performance", which include the following:

Standards of Care

- Assessment
- Diagnosis
- Outcome Identification
- Planning
- Evaluation

Standards of Professional Performance

- Quality of Care
- Performance Appraisal
- Education
- Collegiality

- Ethics
- Collaboration
- Research
- Resource Utilization

Standards of Care

"Standards of Care" describes a competent level of forensic nursing practice as demonstrated by the nursing process, which involves assessment, analysis, outcome identification, implementation, and evaluation. The nursing process encompasses all significant actions taken by forensic nurses in providing services to all clients, and forms the foundation of decision-making. Additional nursing responsibilities for all clients, such as providing culturally and ethnically applicable services, maintaining a safe environment, and planning for continuity of care and services, are embodied within these standards. Therefore, "Standards of Care" delineates services that are provided to all clients of forensic nurses or practitioners.

Standards of Professional Performance

"Standards of Professional Performance" describes a competent level of behavior in the professional role, including activities related to quality of services, performance appraisal, education, collegiality, ethics, collaboration, research, and resource utilization. All forensic nurses are expected to engage in professional role activities appropriate to their education, position, and practice setting. While this is an assumption of all of the "Standards of Professional Performance," the scope of nursing involvement in some professional roles is particularly dependent upon the forensic nurse's education, position, and practice environment. Therefore, some standards or measurement criteria identify a broad range of activities demonstrating compliance with the standard. Where measurement criteria may not apply, delineation of appropriateness will be stated so pertinent discretion is allowed.

While "Standards of Professional Performance" describes roles expected of all forensic nurses, many other responsibilities comprise the hallmarks of this profession. The forensic nurse should be self-directed and purposeful in seeking necessary knowledge and skills to enhance career goals. Other activities, such as membership in a professional nursing organization, certification in a specialty or advanced practice area, and further academic education are desirable methods to enhance the forensic nurse's professionalism.

Criteria

The Scope and Standards of Forensic Nursing Practice include criteria that allow the standards to be measured. Criteria include key indicators of competent forensic nursing practice. For the most part, standards should remain stable over time, as they reflect the philosophical values of the profession. However, criteria should be revised to incorporate advancements in scientific knowledge, practice, research, and technology. Criteria must remain consistent with current forensic nursing practice, which has a theoretical basis but is constantly evolving through the development of new knowledge and incorporation of relevant research findings into aspects of the nursing process.

Assumptions

The *Standards of Clinical Nursing Practice* focuses primarily on the process of providing nursing care and performing professional role activities. These standards apply to all nurses in all areas of clinical practice despite the tremendous variability in environments in which nurses practice. However, it is important to recognize the link between working conditions and the nurse's ability to deliver services. It is the responsibility of employers or health care facilities to provide an appropriate environment for forensic nursing practice.

Although it is the forensic nurse's responsibility to meet these standards, *Scope and Standards of Forensic Nursing Practice* assumes that adequate environmental working conditions and necessary resources are available to support and facilitate the forensic nurse's attainment of these practice standards. Related standards that address the work environment are found in other ANA publications: *Standards for Organized Nursing Services and Responsibilities of Nurse Administrators Across All Settings, Standards for Nursing Staff Development, Standards for Professional Nursing Education, Standards for Continuing Education in Nursing, Code for Nurses with Interpretive Statements, The Scope of Nursing Practice,* and *Education for Participation in Nursing Research.*

These publications and the *Scope and Standards of Forensic Nursing Practice* can be used to determine the resources necessary to provide an adequate work environment. In addition, forensic nurses may benefit from having structural criteria clearly defined within the standards of specialty organizations such as the IAFN.

Several related themes underlie the *Scope and Standards of Forensic Nursing Practice*. Forensic nursing services must be individualized to meet a particular client's unique needs and situation. The forensic nurse also must respect the client's goals and preferences in developing and implementing a plan for services. Given that one of the forensic nurse's primary responsibilities is client education, forensic nurses must provide clients with appropriate information to make informed decisions.

The Scope and Standards of Forensic Nursing Practice also recognizes the forensic nurse's partnership with the client, law enforcement agencies, judicial systems, health care providers, and legal agencies. These standards assume that the forensic nurse may work with other health care providers, law enforcement agencies, judicial systems, or the community in a coordinated manner throughout the process of rendering services to a client. In addition, the involvement of the client, family, and/or significant others is seen as paramount. Of course, the appropriate degree of participation expected of the client, family, or other health care providers must be inferred from the specific clinical environment and the client's unique situation.

Throughout this document, terms such as "appropriate", "pertinent" and "realistic" may be used. It is beyond the scope of a document such as this to account for all possible scenarios that the forensic nurse may encounter in a clinical or community setting. The forensic nurse will need to exercise judgment based on education and experience in determining what is appropriate, pertinent or realistic. Further direction may be available from documents such as guidelines for practice or agency standards, local, state and federal rules, policies, procedures, and protocols.

Purpose

These standards are primarily intended to assist the forensic nurse in providing safe and effective services and to pursue professional development. This document is also designed to:

- Promote the advancement of forensic nursing practice

- Provide an objective base for the development of performance evaluation tools

- Stimulate the development of peer review

- Encourage research to validate forensic nursing practice

- Generate research that may improve forensic practice
- Promote collaboration within the multidisciplinary teams

Summary

The Scope and Standards of Forensic Nursing Practice delineates the professional responsibilities of registered nurses engaged in the specialty of forensic nursing. This publication and nursing practice guidelines could serve as a basis for:

- Quality assurance systems
- Databases
- Regulatory systems
- Health care reimbursement and financing methodologies
- Development and evaluation of nursing service delivery systems and organizational structures
- Certification activities
- Job descriptions and performance appraisals
- Agency policies, procedures and protocols
- Educational offerings.

In order to best serve the public and the forensic nursing profession, forensic nurses must continue efforts to develop standards of practice and practice guidelines. Forensic nurses must examine how standards and practice guidelines can be disseminated and used most effectively to enhance and promote the quality of forensic nursing practice. In addition, standards and practice guidelines must be evaluated on an ongoing basis, with revisions made as necessary. The dynamic nature of the health care environment and the growing body of nursing research provides both the impetus and the means by which forensic nursing will proactively respond to ensure competent practice and promote ongoing professional development and client services.

STANDARDS OF CARE

Standard I. Assessment

The forensic nurse shall provide an accurate assessment, based upon data collected, of the physical and/or psychological issues of the client as related to forensic nursing and/or forensic pathology.

Rationale:	Assessment is a series of systematic, organized, and deliberate actions to identify and obtain data. This assessment provides the data base for the determination of the forensic applications to the client.
Outcome:	Forensic nursing assessment will be done for every client.
Component Standard:	Assessment shall include systematic and pertinent collection of data about the forensic status of the client.

Measurement Criteria

1. Data shall be obtained as determined by the forensic client's immediate needs.

2. The forensic nurse conducts the client assessment within the framework of holistic professional nursing practice which is inclusive of physical and psychological issues achieved within the client interview, observation and assessment.

3. The forensic nurse performs the initial assessment in a timely manner. Ongoing assessments are based on the specific conditions of the forensic issues.

4. The forensic nurse records significant data as appropriate to the nature and extent of the injury, situation or practice area.

5. The forensic nurse follows the chain of custody as indicated.

6. The forensic nurse has ongoing communication regarding significant data as it relates to the appropriate persons throughout the judicial process to facilitate the determination of a forensic diagnosis.

7. The forensic nurse maintains appropriate confidentiality of records where appropriate, while ensuring that all relevant

records are promptly and properly transferred to appropriate persons or institutions as required.

Standard II. Diagnosis

The forensic nurse shall analyze the assessment data to determine a diagnosis pertaining to forensic issues in nursing.

Rationale: Analyses of data provide the basis for planning timely and effective forensic nursing interventions.

Outcome: A systematic process of assessment and data analyses is reflected in appropriate diagnosis and decision making pertaining to forensic issues in nursing.

Component Standard: The forensic nurse shall determine a diagnosis pertaining to forensic nursing issues for whom they provide care and/or services.

Measurement Criteria

1. Diagnosis of forensic issues in nursing are based on identifiable data.

2. The forensic nurse identifies those diagnoses that are consistent with the findings of other forensic health care, law enforcement, and judicial professionals that will facilitate a controlled pathway throughout the judicial process.

3. Diagnoses of forensic assessments in nursing services are consistent with the accepted current bodies of knowledge.

4. The forensic nurse analyzes evidence as appropriate to the area of practice.

Standard III. Outcome Identification

The forensic nurse will identify expected individual outcomes based on the forensic diagnoses of the client.

Rationale: Individualized outcomes provide direction for continuity of services and increased collaborative efforts between all disciplines in the management of clients.

Outcome: An individualized outcome is formulated for every identified diagnosis.

Component   Outcomes shall show that all efforts point toward effective
Standard: services and case coordination and communication in managing forensic clients.

Measurement Criteria

1. Outcomes pertaining to forensic diagnoses are derived from the data.

2. Outcomes are formulated with the client and multidisciplinary team members when possible.

3. Forensic outcomes are attainable in relation to resources available to the client.

4. Forensic outcomes include a time estimate and are documented as measurable goals, if applicable.

Standard IV. Planning

The forensic nurse develops a comprehensive plan of action for the forensic client appropriate to forensic interventions to attain expected outcomes.

Rationale: Safe and effective forensic nursing planning results from active intervention on the part of the forensic nurse as a member of the multidisciplinary team.

Outcome: Evidence of a plan of action exists for forensic issues.

Component   The forensic nurse shall develop and utilize a standard
Standard: plan of action to provide consistency concerning forensic nursing issues.

Measurement Criteria

1. The plan of action identifies and prioritizes the forensic nursing actions, client outcomes, and goals individualized to the forensic nursing issues.

2. The plan of action is developed with a collaborative perspective toward a multidisciplinary approach involving the client, family

members, significant others, health care members, and other disciplines as appropriate by utilizing the client's assessment, interviews, and ongoing evaluations.

3. The plan of action reflects current nursing practice in the forensic nursing arena.

4. The plan of action is documented, as appropriate.

5. The plan of action provides for continuity of care by incorporating forensic teaching and learning principals into the overall plan of care.

Standard V. Implementation

The forensic nurse implements a plan of action based on forensic issues derived from assessment data, nursing diagnoses, and medical diagnoses, when applicable, and scientific knowledge.

Rationale: A base of scientific and conceptual knowledge of nursing science, forensic science and criminal justice in addition to assessment data, provides a foundation for a plan to be implemented in a timely and effective manner.

Outcome: Forensic nursing interventions that reflect a collaborative consideration of the client and significant other, if applicable, are performed in a safe and effective manner. They are consistent with the plan and are documented by written record as applicable.

Component Standard: The forensic nurse shall function independently within the parameters established for professional nursing practice.

Measurement Criteria

1. Documentation reflects competent skill performance and sound judgment in autonomous practice.

2. Standardized care plans pertaining to forensic diagnoses are developed and available for use, if applicable.

3. Modifications and deviations from standard plans of action are noted and documented with supporting data, if applicable.

Component Standard:	The forensic nurse shall function collaboratively within a multidisciplinary team, combining health care with criminal justice and law enforcement agencies and other resources to implement a prescribed regime within the scope of professional nursing practice.

Measurement Criteria

1. The forensic nurse combines biomedical, forensic science, law enforcement and criminal justice training, and education to implement a standardized plan of action.
2. The forensic nurse individualizes the plan of action based on the changing needs of the client, the circumstances or situation, and resources available.

Standard VI. Evaluation

The forensic nurse evaluates and modifies the plan of action to achieve expected outcomes.

Rationale:	Evaluation of forensic nursing services must be based on all outcomes as specified by the goals in the plan of action.
Outcome:	Forensic data are evaluated concurrently and retrospectively to ensure that an acceptable quality of services provided is obtained and maintained.
Component Standard:	Forensic nursing services are evaluated on a continuous basis to determine progress or lack of progress toward goal attainment.

Measurement Criteria

1. Evaluation is systematic and ongoing.
2. Evaluation is used to revise forensic nursing diagnoses, outcomes, and the plan of action as needed.
3. The client's response to intervention of the forensic issues relating to the situation is documented, as appropriate.
4. Revisions in the plan, diagnoses, and outcomes are documented, when appropriate.

5. The client, family members, significant others, and multidisciplinary team members are involved in the evaluation process when appropriate.

STANDARDS OF PROFESSIONAL PERFORMANCE

Standard I. Quality of Care

The forensic nurse systematically evaluates the quality and effectiveness of forensic nursing practice.

Rationale:	Evaluation of forensic nursing practice must be based on observable client outcomes as appropriate to the forensic nurse's position, education, and practice environment to assure quality forensic nursing practice.
Outcome:	Forensic nursing practice is evaluated concurrently and retrospectively to ensure that the quality of practice is maintained.
Component Standard:	A comprehensive plan for quality assurance of forensic nursing practice shall be developed and implemented.

Measurement Criteria

1. Identified problems or deficiencies are carefully reviewed and evaluated to monitor the quality and effectiveness of forensic nursing practice, as appropriate.
2. Data are collected concerning forensic issues in nursing practice and evaluated according to the effectiveness of such practice, as appropriate.
3. Analysis of data is performed to identify opportunities for service improvement, as appropriate.
4. Recommendations are made to improve the quality of forensic nursing services or client outcomes, as appropriate.
5. Activities that enhance the quality of forensic nursing practice are implemented, as appropriate.
6. Policies and procedures reflecting forensic issues in nursing are developed to improve the quality of services provided, as appropriate.

Component   The forensic nurse utilizes the results of quality assurance
Standard: activities to initiate changes in practice.

Measurement Criteria

1. Identification of indicators are used to monitor forensic nursing practice.
2. Standardized plans of care on forensic nursing issues are developed and validated using the results of quality assurance activities as appropriate to the practice area.

Standard II. Performance Appraisal

The forensic nurse evaluates his/her own forensic nursing practice in relation to professional practice standards and relevant statutes and regulations.

Rationale: Safe and effective forensic nursing practice depends on the retention and application of a specified body of knowledge and skills that are developed over time. The primary purpose is to provide a systematic method of documenting and validating specific activities that reflect the forensic dimensions and responsibilities of the forensic nurse.

Outcome: Collaborative and autonomous forensic nursing practice that reflects forensic nursing and research is provided to all forensic clients as appropriate.

Component   The evaluation of individual performance as measured
Standard: against the duties and responsibilities of the forensic nursing job description is a continuous process

Measurement Criteria

1. The forensic nurse engages in performance appraisal on a regular basis identifying areas of strengths as well as areas for professional/practice development.
2. The forensic nurse seeks constructive feedback regarding his/her own practice.
3. The forensic nurse takes action to achieve goals identified during the performance appraisal.

4. The forensic nurse participates in peer review as appropriate.

Standard III. Education

The forensic nurse acquires and maintains current knowledge in forensic nursing practice.

Rationale:	In the process of continuing education, there is not only the responsibility of one's own learning, but also the integration of that learning into daily practice.
Outcome:	The knowledge and skills of forensic nursing are demonstrated and shared in daily practice.
Component Standard:	Forensic nurses shall obtain ongoing education consistent with their level and area of practice.

Measurement Criteria

1. The forensic nurse participates in ongoing educational activities related to clinical knowledge and professional issues.
2. The forensic nurse seeks experience to maintain competence.
3. The forensic nurse seeks knowledge and skills appropriate to the practice setting.

Standard IV. Collegiality

The forensic nurse contributes to the professional development of peers, colleagues and others.

Rationale:	Teaching facilitates the provision of information about the role and responsibilities of forensic nursing and the provision of services provided to forensic clients.
Outcome:	The sharing of learned knowledge with others assists forensic nurses in identifying and meeting their own learning needs to maximize professional development and optimal forensic nursing practice.

Component Standard:	Forensic nurses shall facilitate formal and informal learning experiences for professional peers, colleagues and others.

Measurement Criteria

1. The forensic nurse shares knowledge and skills with colleagues and others in a multidisciplinary educational effort, as appropriate.

2. The forensic nurse provides peers with constructive feedback regarding their practice involving forensic issues.

3. The forensic nurse participates in teaching nursing students and colleagues regarding role responsibilities, policies, procedures and forensic practice, when applicable.

Standard V. Ethics

The forensic nurse's decisions and actions are determined in an ethical manner.

Rationale:	Beliefs in human worth comprise the philosophical foundation on which forensic nursing is based.
Outcome:	The practice of forensic nursing is consistent with the ANA Code of Ethics For Nurses.
Component Standard:	Forensic nurses shall demonstrate an awareness and adherence of local, state and federal laws governing their practice.

Measurement Criteria

1. The forensic nurse follows chain of custody when obtaining evidence and/or specimens for forensic purposes.

2. The forensic nurse maintains and preserves any evidence collected.

3. The forensic nurse follows chain of custody when turning over evidentiary material.

4. The forensic nurse reports appropriately according to local, state and federal mandates.

5. The forensic nurse obtains appropriate informed consent for evidence collection, procedures, treatment, or photography as appropriate.

6. The forensic nurse informs clients of their legal rights as required, in collaboration with appropriate individuals.

7. The forensic nurse maintains client confidentiality, where appropriate.

8. The forensic nurse seeks available resources related to legal and ethical issues for the forensic client.

Component Standard: The forensic nurse delivers services in a non-judgmental and non-discriminatory manner that is sensitive to client diversity.

Measurement Criteria

1. The forensic nurse respects the individuality and human worth of forensic clients regardless of age, sexual orientation, socio-economic status, cultural or ethical background or spiritual beliefs.

2. The forensic nurse delivers services in a manner that respects the dignity, confidentiality and privacy of forensic clients, where appropriate.

Standard VI. Collaboration

The forensic nurse collaborates with the forensic client, family members, significant others and multidisciplinary team members.

Rationale: The forensic nurse is non-judgmental and facilitates communication between the client, family members, significant others, and the legal and judicial system.

Outcome: The forensic nurse promotes open communication among multidisciplinary team members to ensure the occurrence of effective forensic interventions.

Component
Standard:

The forensic nurse communicates with the client, family members, significant others, and multidisciplinary team members regarding services provided.

Measurement Criteria

1. The forensic nurse involves the client, family and significant others as appropriate, in decision making processes related to the forensic issues.

Component
Standard:

Forensic nurses participate in formal and informal investigative methodology related to forensic issues and the community.

Measurement Criteria

1. The forensic nurse collaborates with other members of the multidisciplinary team as appropriate, to provide services throughout the judicial system.

2. The forensic nurse collaborates with those practicing within the judicial system as necessary, to ensure that judicial procedure is maintained within the scope of the issues involving the client.

3. Diagnoses of forensic issues are documented and reflect a collaborative approach to the delivery of services.

4. The forensic nurse communicates with multidisciplinary team members as appropriate regarding forensic issues.

5. Collaboration with multidisciplinary team members is done to evaluate forensic nursing practice.

6. The forensic nurse communicates with and participates as a member of a multidisciplinary team

Standard VII. Research

The forensic nurse recognizes, values and utilizes research as a method to further forensic nursing practice.

Rationale:

Research is necessary to develop a body of validated forensic nursing knowledge on which forensic nursing is based.

| *Outcome:* | The forensic nurse makes improvements in the quality of forensic nursing practice administered. |

| *Component Standard:* | The forensic nurse shall utilize those interventions substantiated by research to improve forensic nursing practice. |

Measurement Criteria

1. The forensic nurse utilizes current knowledge of research in forensic nursing practice.

2 The forensic nurse implements changes in practice based upon forensic nursing research.

| *Component Standard:* | The forensic nurse participates in research activities as appropriate to the practitioner's position, education and practice environment. |

Measurement Criteria

1. The forensic nurse possesses the skills necessary to conduct research, as appropriate.

2. The forensic nurse participates in ongoing projects by identification of problems pertaining to forensic issues.

3. The forensic nurse collaborates with colleagues in their research within the practice setting.

Standard VIII. Resource Utilization

The forensic nurse considers factors related to safety, effectiveness, and cost in planning and delivering forensic services.

| *Rationale:* | Safe and effective forensic nursing practice results from active planning on the part of the forensic nurse in identifying and securing cost effective resources available to address forensic issues. |

| *Outcome:* | Evidence of planning and delivery of safe and effective forensic nursing practice is documented. |

Component   The forensic nurse considers factors related to safety, effec-
Standard: tiveness, and cost, based on the needs of the forensic client.

Measurement Criteria

1.   The forensic nurse evaluates forensic nursing practice for safety
        and cost, with a collaborative outlook toward a multidisciplinary
        approach involving the client, significant others, and other disci-
        plines as appropriate.

2.   The forensic nurse delegates services based on the needs of the
        client and the knowledge and skills of the provider.

3.   The forensic nurse makes modifications to services provided as
        necessary in securing appropriate resources for the client.

BIBLIOGRAPHY

American Nurses Association. 1991. *Standards of clinical nursing practice*, Washington, DC: Author.

American Nurses Association. 1995. *Nursing's social policy statement*, Washington, DC: Author.

American Nurses Association. 1987. *The scope of nursing practice*, Washington, DC: Author.

American Nurses Association. 1996. *Standards of oncology nursing practice*, Washington, DC: American Nurses Association and The Oncology Nursing Society.

Emergency Nurses Association. 1991. *Standards of emergency nursing practice* (2nd ed.). St. Louis: C.V. Mosby Company.

Gordon, M. 1987. *Nursing diagnosis: Process and application* (2nd ed.) St. Louis: Mosby Year Book, Inc.

Joint Commission of Accreditation of Healthcare Organizations. 1996. *Accreditation manual for hospitals*. Chicago: Author.

Lynch, Virginia. 1993. Forensic aspects of health care: New roles, new responsibilities. *Journal of Psychosocial Nursing* 31(11).

GLOSSARY

Assessment: A systematic, dynamic process by which the forensic nurse, through interaction with the client, significant others, the community, health care providers, law enforcement agencies and judicial systems, collects and analyzes data about the client. Data may include the following dimensions: physical, psychological, sociocultural, spiritual, cognitive, functional abilities, developmental, economic, and life-style.

Client: Recipient of forensic nursing services. When the client is an individual, the focus may be the health state, problems or needs of a single person. When the client is a family or group, the focus may be on the health state of the unit as a whole or the reciprocal effects of an individual's health state on the other members of the unit. When the client is a community, the focus is on personal and environmental health and safety, and the risk factors of population groups. Nursing services to clients may be directed to disease or injury prevention, health and safety promotion, health restoration, health maintenance, crime prevention, evidence collection and preservation, and expert testimony. The client may also be the decedent, who will be at the focus of a death investigation.

Continuity of care: An interdisciplinary process that includes clients, family members, significant others and multidisciplinary team members in the development of a coordinated plan of service. This process facilitates the client's transition between settings, based on needs and available resources.

Criteria: Relevant, measurable indicators of the standards of forensic nursing practice.

Diagnosis: A judgment about the response to actual or potential conditions or needs. Diagnoses provide the basis for determination of a plan of services to achieve expected outcomes.

Evaluation: The process of determining both the progress toward the attainment of expected outcomes and the effectiveness of forensic nursing services.

Forensic nursing: The application of the forensic aspects of health care combined with the bio-psychological education of the registered nurse in the scientific investigation and treatment of trauma and/or death related medical-legal issues.

Guidelines: Describes a process of client service management that has the potential of improving the quality of services provided and consumer decision making. Guidelines are systematically developed statements based on available scientific evidence and expert opinion.

Nursing: The diagnosis and treatment of human responses to actual or potential health problems.

Outcomes: Measurable, expected focused goals.

Plan of action: Comprehensive outline of services delivered to attain expected outcomes.

Planning: May include any or all of these activities: intervening, delegating or coordinating. The client, significant other, agency, service organization, law enforcement agency, judicial system, or health care provider may be designated to implement interventions within the plan of services.

Providers: Individuals, service organizations, agencies and professionals with special expertise who provide services or assistance to clients.

Significant others: Family members and/or those significant to the client.

Standard: Authoritative statement enunciated and promulgated by the profession by which the quality of practice, service, or education can be judged.

Standards of care: Authoritative statements that describe a competent level of forensic nursing practice demonstrated through assessment, diagnosis, outcome identification, planning, implementation, and evaluation as appropriate to the practice setting.

Standards of forensic nursing practice: Authoritative statements that describe a level of service or performance common to the profession of forensic nursing by which the quality of forensic nursing practice can be judged. Standards of practice include both standards of care and standards of professional performance.

Standards of professional performance: Authoritative statements that describe a competent level of behavior in the professional role, including activities related to quality of service, performance appraisal, education, collegiality, ethics, collaboration, research, and resource utilization.

Victim: The victim is one that is acted upon and usually adversely affected by an outside incident. In forensic nursing, the victim may be the client, the decedent, the perpetrator, the family, significant others, the suspect, the accused and/or falsely accused, the community and/or the public in general.

INDEX

An index entry preceded by the bracketed calendar year [1997] indicates an entry from *Scope and Standards of Forensic Nursing*. That 1997 publication is included, for reference only, in this edition as Appendix A: its content is not current and is of historical significance only.

Patients in forensic nursing
  characteristics, 3–4
  advocacy for, 2, 13, 16, 28
  defined, 51
  [1997] 95
diversity of patient population, 4–5
See also Perpetrators ... ; Victims in
  forensic nursing
Peer review, 10, 16
  collegiality and, 52
  in professional practice evaluation, 14,
  35
  defined, 51
Performance appraisal, [1997] 87–88
  See also Professional practice evaluation
Perpetrators in forensic nursing
  as co-focus with victims, xi, 1, 2, 4, 6,
  12, 15
  defined, 51
  development of focus, 6
  See also Victims in forensic nursing
Plan (defined), 52
  See also Planning
Plan of action (defined), 52
Planning, 1
  consultation to influence, 31
  evaluation and, 33–34
  expected outcomes from, 3
  coordinating implementation of plan,
  29
  implementation of plan, 28
  resource utilization and, 45–46
  standard of practice, 26–27
  [1997] as standard of care, 82–83
Populations as focus of forensic nursing,
  1, 2, 4, 5, 7, 11, 13, 15, 16, 17
  See also Public health
Practice characteristics of forensic
  nursing, 7–10
  collaboration, 40
  [1997] 90–91
Practice settings, 7–11
  roles and, 3–6
  systems intersecting, 3–4, 53
Prescriptive authority and treatment
  in advanced practice, 15, 32
  standard of practice, 32

Preventive focus of forensic nursing, xi,
  2, 5, 6, 7, 10, 12, 15, 16, 18
Professional organizations in forensic
  nursing
  American Nurses Association (ANA),
  x–xi, 16, 77
  Canadian Nurses Association, x, xi
  International Association of Forensic
  Nurses (IAFN), 6
Professional performance. See Standards
  of professional performance
Professional practice evaluation, x
  peer review and, 14, 35
  standard of professional performance,
  38
  See also Peer review
Providers
  defined, 52
  [1997] 96
Psychiatric nurse, 9–10
Public health and forensic nursing, xi, 2,
  4, 5, 10, 13, 17
  violence as public health issue (1984), 6

Q
Quality of care, 10
  [1997] 86–87
  defined, 52
Quality of practice, 10, 11, 45
  standard of professional performance,
  35–36

R
Referrals and forensic nurses, 32, 40
Registered nurse (RN), 7
Regulatory issues. See Legal, regulatory,
  and statutory issues
Research, 1, 3, 10, 18
  standard of professional performance,
  43–44
  [1997] 91–92
Resource utilization
  community resources, 4, 28, 29, 45
  organizational resources, 45, 46
  standard of professional performance,
  45–46
  [1997] 92–93

Risk management nurse, 8–9
RN (registered nurse), 7
Role differentiation in forensic nursing
  psychiatric nurse, 9–10
  risk management nurse, 8–9
  sexual assault nurse examiner (SANE),
    5–6

S
Safety and forensic nursing
  quality of practice and, 35–36
  resource utilization and, 45–46
  [1997] 92–93
SANE (sexual assault nurse examiner),
    5–6, 14–15
  See also Sexual assault and abuse
Scientific findings. *See* Evidence-based
  practice; Research
Scope of forensic nursing practice, *x–xi*,
    1–19
  function of, 1
Scope of nursing practice, *x–xi*, 52
  function of, *ix*
Scope of Nursing Practice (ICN), *xi*, 77
Self-care (nurses) as ethical element of
  practice, 41
Self-care (patients) in health teaching
  and promotion, 30
Self-harm and self-injury, 7, 9
Self monitoring. *See* Self-care
Sexual assault and abuse, 5–6, 9
  sexual assault nurse examiner (SANE),
    5–6, 14–15
  See also Victims in forensic nursing
Significant other
  defined, 52
  [1997] 96
Skills and abilities of forensic nurses.
    See Knowledge base of forensic
    nursing
Specialization in forensic nursing, 4
  [1997] 70
Standardized languages in planning,
    26
Standards (nursing)
  defined, 52

function of, *ix–x*, 21
legal standard of care and, *ix–x*, 21
Standards of care for forensic nursing
    [1997]
  assessment 80–81
  defined, 96
  development of, 74
  diagnosis, 81
  evaluation, 84–85
  implementation, 83–84
  outcome identification, 81–82
  planning, 82–83
  See also Standards of practice for
    forensic nursing
*Standards for Continuing Education in
    Nursing* (ANA), 77
Standards of forensic nursing practice,
    defined, [1997] 96
Standards of nursing care (defined),
    [1997] 76
Standards for Nursing Staff Development
    (ANA), 77
*Standards for Organized Nursing
    Services and Responsibilities of
    Nurse Administrators Across All
    Settings* (ANA), 77
Standards of practice for forensic nursing
  assessment, 23
  consultation, 31
  coordination of care, 29
  defined, 52
  development of, *ix–xi*
  diagnosis, 24
  evaluation, 33–34
  function of, 21
  health teaching and health
    promotion, 30
  implementation, 28
  outcomes identification, 25
  planning, 26–27
  prescriptive authority and treatment, 32
  role of standards, [1997] 74
  See also Standards of care for forensic
    nursing; *Each standard*
*Standards for Professional Nursing
    Education* (ANA), 77